Ana Kleiner
Manuela Galli
Ricardo M. L. Barros

The Required Coefficient of Friction in Normal and Pathological Gait

AF138221

Ana Kleiner
Manuela Galli
Ricardo M. L. Barros

The Required Coefficient of Friction in Normal and Pathological Gait

LAP LAMBERT Academic Publishing

Impressum / Imprint

Bibliografische Information der Deutschen Nationalbibliothek: Die Deutsche Nationalbibliothek verzeichnet diese Publikation in der Deutschen Nationalbibliografie; detaillierte bibliografische Daten sind im Internet über http://dnb.d-nb.de abrufbar.
Alle in diesem Buch genannten Marken und Produktnamen unterliegen warenzeichen-, marken- oder patentrechtlichem Schutz bzw. sind Warenzeichen oder eingetragene Warenzeichen der jeweiligen Inhaber. Die Wiedergabe von Marken, Produktnamen, Gebrauchsnamen, Handelsnamen, Warenbezeichnungen u.s.w. in diesem Werk berechtigt auch ohne besondere Kennzeichnung nicht zu der Annahme, dass solche Namen im Sinne der Warenzeichen- und Markenschutzgesetzgebung als frei zu betrachten wären und daher von jedermann benutzt werden dürften.

Bibliographic information published by the Deutsche Nationalbibliothek: The Deutsche Nationalbibliothek lists this publication in the Deutsche Nationalbibliografie; detailed bibliographic data are available in the Internet at http://dnb.d-nb.de.
Any brand names and product names mentioned in this book are subject to trademark, brand or patent protection and are trademarks or registered trademarks of their respective holders. The use of brand names, product names, common names, trade names, product descriptions etc. even without a particular marking in this work is in no way to be construed to mean that such names may be regarded as unrestricted in respect of trademark and brand protection legislation and could thus be used by anyone.

Coverbild / Cover image: www.ingimage.com

Verlag / Publisher:
LAP LAMBERT Academic Publishing
ist ein Imprint der / is a trademark of
OmniScriptum GmbH & Co. KG
Heinrich-Böcking-Str. 6-8, 66121 Saarbrücken, Deutschland / Germany
Email: info@lap-publishing.com

Herstellung: siehe letzte Seite /
Printed at: see last page
ISBN: 978-3-659-71604-1

Zugl. / Approved by: Campinas, University of Campinas, Diss., 2015

The Required Coefficient of Friction in Normal and Pathological Gait.

Ana Kleiner, Manuela Galli and Ricardo M.L. Barros.

To my family for all the love and support.

This work was supported by two scholarships granted by **CAPES Foundation, Ministry of Education of Brazil**. The first was the institutional PhD scholarship that supported the part of this thesis performed in Brazil at Laboratory of Instrumentation for Biomechanics, College of Physical Education, University of Campinas, Campinas – Brazil, and supervised by Prof. Ricardo M. L. Barros, and the second was the PDSE scholarship (BEX 11241/13-6). Thanks to the PDSE scholarship, t this thesis was also developed at "Luigi Divieti" Posture and Movement Analysis Laboratory, Department of Electronics, Information and Bioengineering, Politecnico di Milano, Milan, Italy, supervised by Prof. PhD. Manuela Galli.

Summary

Introduction

Slips and falls are recognized as important occupational safety concerns and considered to be among the major causes of unintentional injury (Kemmlert and Lundholm, 2001; Layne and Pollack, 2004; Leamon and Murphy, 1995). Falls precipitated by slipping are of major concern (Courtney et al., 2001). Lloyd and Stevenson (1992) reported that slips and trips cause 67% and 32% of falls sustained by the elderly and young, respectively.

Understanding what causes slip-precipitated pedestrian accidents is challenging because of the multiple, interacting environmental and human factors involved. Among the environmental factors are properties of the flooring (e.g. surface roughness); human factors include gait, the health of the sensory systems (e.g. vision, proprioception, somatosensation, and vestibular) and neurological pathologies such as Stroke and Parkinson's Disease (PD).

Hemiplegia is one of the most common impairments after stroke and contributes significantly to reduce gait performance. Although the majority of stroke patients achieve independent gait, many do not reach a walking level that enable them to perform all their daily activities (Flansbjer et al., 2005). Moreover, after completing standard rehabilitation, approximately 50%-60% of stroke patients still experience some degree of motor impairment, and approximately 50% are at least partly dependent in activities-of-daily-living (Schaechter, 2004). Fall incidence rates between 23% and 50% have been reported in studies of people with chronic stroke (6 months post-stroke – Jorgensen et al., 2002; Lamb et al., 2003; Hyndman et al., 2002; Hyndman et al., 2003). This rate is much higher than rates reported for older community-dwelling adults without stroke (11%–30% - Bogle et al., 1996; Graafmans et al., 1996). Over half of all reported falls occurred indoors during walking activities (Jorgensen et al., 2002; Hyndman et al., 2002).

Patients with PD have high risk of falling, even compared to age-matched controls. In a community based sample of 63 patients with PD, Ashburn et al. (2001) found that 40% had

6

experienced one or more falls in the previous 12 months. In a 6-month, prospective study, Bloem at al. (2001) observed that 51% of PD subjects with moderately advanced disease fell at least once while only 15% of age-matched control subjects fell. Gray and Hildebrand (2000) observed that 59% of PD subjects fell during a 3-month period. In a 1-year prospective study, Wood et al. (2002) reported that 68% of the PD subjects had at least one fall.

As described, both pathologies provide abnormal gait pattern and the most significant consequence of this are falls. Falls may lead to injuries, hip fractures, fear of falling, and restriction of activities that in turn contribute to institutionalization, loss of independence and increased mortality (Schaafsma et al., 2003; Harris et al., 2005).

Friction plays an important role in falls (Chang et al., 2001). One ground reaction forces (GRF) measure that has been used to quantify and understand the biomechanics of slips has been the ratio of shear to normal GRF components. During normal locomotion on dry surfaces, i.e. no-slip conditions, this ratio has been described as the Required Coefficient of Friction (RCOF) (Redfern and Andres, 1984; Rhoades and Miller, 1988; Grönqvist et al., 1999).

Perkins (1978) observed the GRF exerted between the shoe and ground in the normal gait cycle, and calculated the ratio of horizontal to vertical foot forces (Fh/Fv). According to this author, the ratio (Fh/Fv) has been used to identify where in the gait cycle a slip is most likely to occur (slip initiation). In the Figure 1 the horizontal force component Fh and the vertical force component Fv are illustrated.

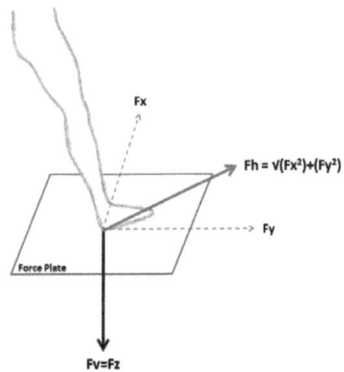

Figure 1. Ground reaction forces generated during walking are used to calculate the COF. Legend: Fx = lateral ground reaction force; Fy = anterior-posterior ground reaction force; Fz = vertical ground reaction force.

There are a variety of pedestrian gaits (e.g. level walking, load carrying, walking up ramps, walking velocity) that have different levels of RCOF to prevent slip. Thus, biomechanical analysis of gait is potentially a valuable tool in the reduction of slip-induced fall accidents because it can elucidate the conditions that may be hazardous to pedestrians (Redfern et al., 2001).

The main goal of this thesis is to analyze the RCOF on elderly, stroke and PD gait. More specifically, this thesis aiming to: (a) to investigate the effect of flooring on RCOF during the barefoot gait considering age (middle-aged versus elderly adults) and gender aspects; (b) to investigate the effect of flooring in foot/floor friction during stroke gait considering this population's lowers limb asymmetry (affected and unaffected lower limbs); (c) to analyze the RCOF instantaneous curves of these patients during the barefoot gait; and, (d) to characterize the RCOF curves of patients with PD during barefoot gait.

This thesis is presented in six chapters. In the First Chapter the literature review of Tribology (the study of friction) and the RCOF during the gait are presented. The Second Chapter discusses the methodology to calculate the RCOF based on the ground reaction forces. The Third and Forty Chapters present the effects of flooring on RCOF during elderly and stroke gait. Finally, the instantaneous RCOF curves analysis in persons with stroke and PD are discuss in the Fifth and Sixth Chapters.

Chapter 1. Friction: Tribology and Human Gait.

1.1. Introduction

In the human gait the timing and placement of successive steps must be continuously adjusted in order to maintain dynamic balance of the body (Nashner, 1980). A prompt and accurate human response to this flow of information appears to be a necessary propensity for slip/fall avoidance. A dynamic interplay needs to exist between the sensory systems (vision, vestibular organ, and proprioception) that control posture, gait and balance (Grönqvist et al., 1999; Redfern et al., 2001), and the friction between shoes/feet and surfaces (Chang et al., 2001a, b).

The aim of this Chapter is to review the concepts of Tribology in human gait.

1.2. Definition and History of Tribology

The expression Tribology originates from the Greek word *tribos*, which means rubbing (Persson, 2000). Tribology is the study of friction, wear, lubrication, and the design of bearings; the science of interacting surfaces in relative motion. More specifically, Tribology is the science and technology of interacting surfaces in relative motion and of related subjects and practices (Bhushan, 2002). The nature and consequence of the interactions that take place at the interface control its friction, wear, and lubrication behavior. During these interactions, forces are transmitted, mechanical energy is converted, the physical and the chemical nature, including surface topography, of the interacting materials are altered. Understanding the nature of these interactions and solving the technological problems associated with the interfacial phenomena constitute the essence of Tribology (Bhushan, 2002).

More than 400.000 years ago, our hominid ancestors used friction when they chipped stone tools. Friction was essential when the Neanderthals by 200.000 B.C. succeeded in generating fire by rubbing wood on wood and by striking together flint stones (Israelachvili, 1995; Bhushan, 2002). Early civilizations, like the Sumerian and Egyptian, discovered the usefulness of lubricants in improving the performance of chariots and in facilitating transport by sleds. Figure 2 shows a painting from the tomb of Tehuti-Hetep at El-Beshed dated at about 1880 B.C., where the Egyptian method of moving stone statues is illustrated. The painting shows that the statue is moved by means of a sled, without the aid of rollers or levers. A most interesting detail in the painting is a man standing and pouring lubricant from a jar onto the ground immediately in front of the sled (Israelachvili, 1995; Bhushan, 2002).

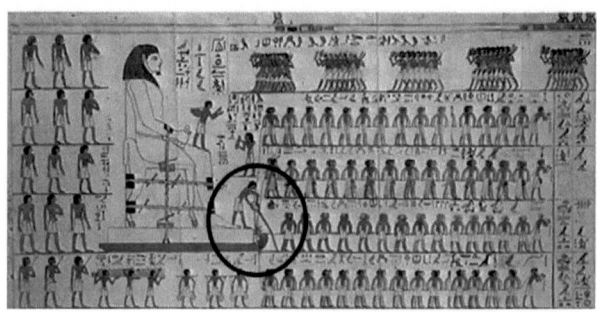

Figure 2. A painting from the tomb of Tehuti-Hetep at El-Beshed (dated about 1880 B.C.), illustrating the transportation of an Egyptian colossus.

Leonardo da Vinci (1452-1519) can be named as the father of modern Tribology (Bhushan, 2002). He studied an incredible manifold of tribological subtopics such as: friction, wear, bearing materials, plain bearings, lubrication systems, gears, screw-jacks, and rolling-element bearings. One Hundred and Fifty years before Amontons' Laws of Friction were introduced da Vinci had already recorded them in his manuscripts: the Codex Atlanticus and the Codex Arundel. The Figure 3 presents some of da Vinci's studies about friction. Hidden or lost for centuries, da Vinci's manuscripts were read in Spain a quarter of a millennium later.

In 1495 da Vinci deduced that the friction force was a fraction of the normal force, that is presented in Equation 1:

$$F = \mu N \tag{1}$$

Where F is the friction force (tangential), μ is the coefficient of friction (constant), N is the normal component of the contact force between the contacting bodies. Moreover, da Vinci deduced the two basic laws of friction: (a) The friction force is dependent on the force pressing bodies together; (b) The friction force is independent of the apparent area of contact (Bhushan, 2002).

Leonard Euler, in 1725, established that the μ was different for static conditions (μ^s) for dynamic or kinetic conditions (μ^k) (Bhushan, 2002). He found that (Equation 2):

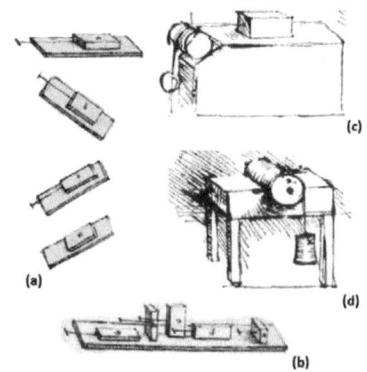

Figure 3. Leonardo da Vinci's studies of friction. Sketches from the Codex Atlanticus and the Codex Arundel showing experiments to determine: (a) the force of friction between horizontal and inclined planes; (b) the influence of apparent contact area upon the force friction; (c) the force of friction on a horizontal plane by means of a pulley; (d) the friction torque on a roller and half bearing.

$$\mu^s > \mu^k \tag{2}$$

Years later, in 1775, Charles A. Coulomb affirmed that kinetic friction (μ^k) is independent of the sliding speed.

In summary, the three classical friction laws were discovered by da Vinci and Guillaume Amontons, respectively, and were summarized much later by Charles-Augustin Coulomb, who also contributed the third friction law (Bhushan, 2002). The three laws of friction are:

11

1ˢᵗ Friction Law: The force of friction is directly proportional to the applied load (da Vinci –
Amontons);

2ⁿᵈ Friction Law: The force of friction is independent of the apparent area of contact (da Vinci –
Amontons);

3ʳᵈ Friction Law: Kinetic friction is independent of the sliding velocity (Coulomb's).

These three laws were attributed to dry friction only, as it has been well known since ancient
times that lubrication modifies the tribological properties significantly.

1.3. Theory of Friction

Friction is the resistance acting against two surfaces lying against each other such as to oppose
their sliding relative to each other. It is one of the oldest problems in physics and it is of great practical
importance in many industrial operations (Bhushan, 1999). Minimizing friction is essential for the
energetic efficiency of many processes and it has become a crucial factor in small-scale moving
devices, such as miniature motors, magnetic storage devices and aerospace components. Friction is
not however just a nuisance. Without friction there would be no violin music and it would be
impossible to walk (Bhushan, 1999). The theory of friction presented here is described in the level of
detail required for a basic understanding. Particular attention is paid to the properties of viscoelastic
materials, since these are characteristic for elements of the friction system.

The term static friction describes the friction of the system at rest. Dynamic friction is defined
by the dynamic friction force F. This is the force required to maintain a body in a constant state of
motion.

Friction is the resistance to motion during sliding or rolling that is experienced when a solid
body moves tangentially over another with which it is in contact. The resistive tangential force, which

acts in a direction directly opposite to the direction of motion is called the friction force (Bönig, 1996). The coefficient of friction is the quotient obtained when the friction force is divided by the normal force acting on the contact.

1.3.1. State and components of friction

Friction may occur in a number of states, like: solid friction, semi-fluid friction, fluid friction and air friction (Bönig, 1996). The friction that occurs with direct contact between the friction counterparts it is describes as solid friction (Figure 4a). By contrast, fluid friction arises when the friction counterparts are completely separated by a fluid film which is not penetrated by roughness peaks (Figure 4b). Where the surfaces of the friction counterparts come into partial contact with each other, the friction assumes the form of semi-fluid friction (Figure 4c). The state of air friction, in which the friction counterparts are fully separated by gaseous phase, is not relevant to the slip resistance, owing to the very high relative velocities which it requires (Figure 4d).

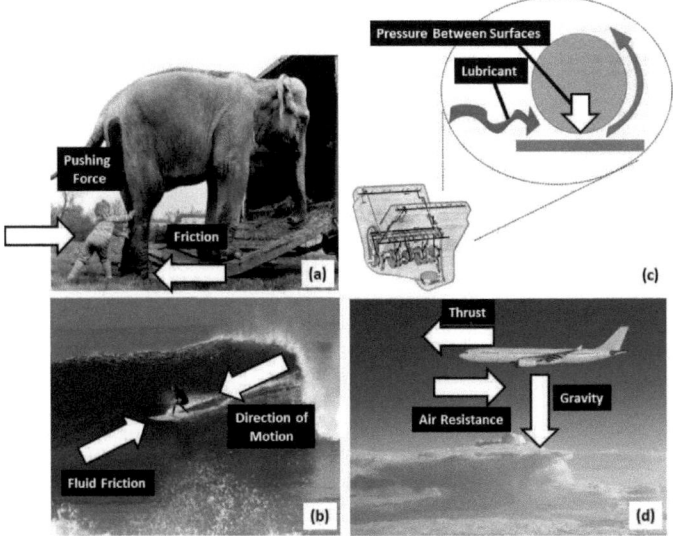

Figure 4. The states of friction: (a) solid friction; (b) fluid friction; (c) semi-fluid friction; and, (d) air friction.

13

The solid friction is composed of three components which arise as a result of adhesion, deformation and cohesion of the friction counterparts (Bönig, 1996; Bhushan, 2002).

(a) Adhesion component: adhesion refers to the forces of molecular attraction acting on the surface between two bodies in very close proximity to each other. The adhesion force component of the frictional force is equal to the tractive force which is required to overcome the attraction forces by shearing of the molecular bonds. The adhesion component of the solid friction in particular rises where the surfaces are smooth (Bönig, 1996).

All surfaces of solid bodies are rough on an atomic scale. For nominally smooth surfaces the surface roughness manifests itself on different scales, on the micrometer scale, on the submicrometer scale and eventually at the atomic level. When two surfaces are brought into contact, the real area of contact is only a small fraction of the apparent area of contact. This is because the surface roughness causes contact to occur only at discrete spots, sometimes referred to as junctions. The sum of the junction areas constitutes the real area of contact. The real area of contact is dependent on the surface texture, on the material properties and on the interfacial loading conditions (Bönig, 1996).

When two surfaces in contact move relative to each other, the friction force is contributed to the adhesion between the junctions and other sources of surface interactions. Upon loading, contact between the two surfaces will initially occur only at a few points to support the load. Due to the small size of the real contact area the stresses at the contact regions may exceed the yield strength of the material, and this will cause the surface to deform at the contact regions (Bowden and Tabor, 1964). The mode of deformation is elastic, elastic-plastic, viscoelastic or viscoplastic. As the normal load increases, a larger number of asperities on the two surfaces come into contact, and existing contact areas grow to support the load (Bhushan, 1999; Tsukruk et al., 1996).

(b) Deformation component: deformation friction is also termed hysteresis friction. The force acting upon a viscoelastic body is associated with a deformation which, when the force is removed, causes less energy to be released than was applied. This hysteresis loss is equal to the work of friction that is converted in the process into heat. For the relative displacement of two bodies against each other,

14

a certain deformation friction force must be generated in order for the work of friction to be performed. The magnitude of deformation force component is influenced by the viscoelasticity of the material and by the surface roughness. On rough surfaces, the deformation friction force may be presumed to constitute a large component of the solid frictional force (Bönig, 1996).

(c) Cohesion component: whereas the above friction components are attributable to external friction, cohesion is the internal friction caused by the shearing off of parts of a substance (Bönig, 1996). Abrasion and wear are clear indicators of the action of a cohesion force. The cohesion force is however of only minor importance, since according to Schallamch (1963) it accounts for less than 2% of the solid frictional force.

1.3.2. Friction of Viscoelastic Materials

Viscoelastic is the property of materials that exhibit both viscous and elastic features when undergoing deformation. The conventional laws of friction apply only in part to viscoelastic materials, from which the majority of shoe soles and many floor coverings are manufactured, as well our skin.

In viscoelastic substances the coefficient of friction is dependent of the surface pressure. Moreover, a dependency upon the sliding velocity exits for viscoelastic materials. Wieder (1988) describes the influence of the sliding velocity upon the adhesion and hysteresis force and upon the fluid friction. According to Kummer (1966), the influences of these two components are superimposed in solid friction. In the low sliding-velocity range, a maximum coefficient of friction is attained by the adhesion force component. At higher velocities, the hysteresis component gains in influence and the coefficient of friction raises continually. The material has a major influence upon the friction of viscoelastic materials (Bönig, 1996).

1.4. Friction in Human Gait

The Figure 5 illustrates the force relationship during the human walking. The force acting at the ground surface is divided into a vertical force component, the normal force N, and the horizontal force component acting at ground level, F. This tangential force F is further subdivided into a tangential force component in the direction of walking, F_Y and a tangential force component perpendicular to the direction of walking, F_X. The force components acting upon the ground give rise to reaction forces of equal magnitude. Owing to the ground geometry, the normal force is transmitted positively, the tangential force non-positively. The tangential force is thus opposed by a frictional force F_R of the same magnitude. The transfer momentum is possible only frictionally, at the ground level, and is of secondary relevance to slip resistance (Bönig, 1996).

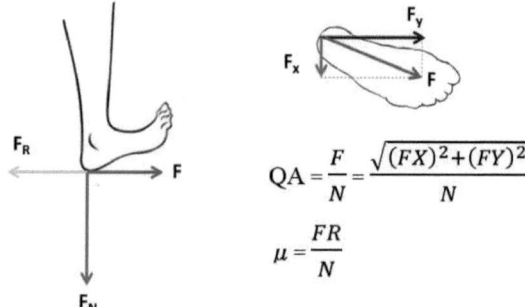

$$QA = \frac{F}{N} = \frac{\sqrt{(FX)^2 + (FY)^2}}{N}$$

$$\mu = \frac{FR}{N}$$

Figure 5. Force relationships during the human horizontal normal walking (modified, nased upon paper04). Legend: N = normal force; F_R = dynamic frictional force; F = tangential force; F_X = tangential force perpendicular to the direction of walking; F_Y = tangential force in direction of walking; Q_A = requirement quotient; μ = coefficient of friction.

The instantaneous requirements upon the frictional system brought about by the walk are described by placing the tangential force in relation to the normal force. The resulting parameter Q_A is referred to as the requirement quotient, and can be compared directly to the coefficient of friction (μ), since the latter is produced by division of the frictional force by the normal force (Bönig, 1996).

During the gait, the required coefficient of friction (RCOF) is the friction required at the shoe and floor. It is typically measured on dry surfaces with a force plate and it is obtained by dividing the component of the measured ground reaction force tangent to the floor surface by the normal component during a step (Redfern et al., 2001).

The RCOF are typically characterized by two peaks. The first peak occurs at the end of the loading phase (about 20% into stance) as full body weight is transferred to the supporting foot, while the second peak occurs later in stance (about 90%) just prior to the beginning of the toe-off phase. The anterior-posterior shear forces exhibit a biphasic, symmetrical shape with the first major peak in the forward direction attributed to the loading dynamics, while the second maximum in the rearward direction happens as the heel rotates off the floor pushing back the toes to start the toe-off phase.

These two phases appear to be two different directional slips during a normal walking step: forward and backward slip during the weight acceptance and backward slip during the toe-off phase (Redfern et al., 2001); it is likely that the forward slip at the landing phase would be the most dangerous due to the body weight being progressively transferred onto the slipping foot. The forward momentum of the body would make it difficult to remove the weight from that foot to regain balance and continued slip would be likely to result in a completely irrecoverable situation.

Previous studies suggested that RCOF is associated with several gait parameters (Copper et al., 2008;Gronqvist et al., 2001; Kim et al., 2005; Lockhart et al., 2003; Redfern et al., 2001). For example, walking velocity directly affects the magnitude of shear force (Fh), and therefore also has a direct effect on RCOF (Kim et al., 2005). Initial gait characteristic such as slower transitional acceleration of the whole-body center of mass may affect RCOF due to the increase in horizontal foot force (Kim et al., 2005; Lockhart et al., 2003). Studies also suggested that changes in step length may influence RCOF (Cooper et al., 2008).

The force interactions between the shoe and floor are probably the most critical biomechanical parameters in slips and falls. If the shear forces generated during a particular step exceed the frictional capabilities of the shoe/floor interface, then a slip is inevitable. Thus, an understanding of the forces at the shoe/floor interface is important. In the next chapter the methodology to evaluate the RCOF during the gait is exposed.

Chapter 2. How to calculate the RCOF with a force plate?

In the Chapter 1 the concepts of Tribology and coefficient of friction in human gait were discussed. Continuing the previous chapter, this chapter presents the methodology used to calculate the RCOF with a force platform.

In this Chapter the methodology used to calculate the instantaneous RCOF as well the RCOF is detailed presented.

2.1. The Force Plate

As we discussed in the previous Chapter the RCOF is typically measured on dry surfaces with a force plate. The force plate consists of a board in which some (often four) force sensors of load cell type or piezoelectric are distributed to measure the three ground reaction force (GRF) components, Fx, Fy and Fz, the lateral, the anterior-posterior, and the vertical directions, respectively (Figure 6).

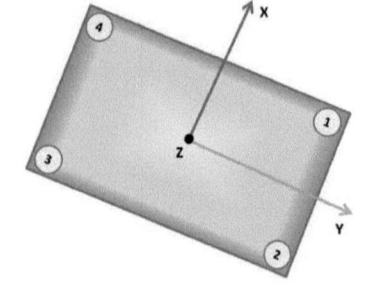

PARAMETER	CALCULATION	DESCRIPTION
Fx	= fx12 + fx34	Lateral Force
Fy	= fy14 + fy23	Anterior-Posterior Force
Fz	= fz1 + fz2 + fz3 + fz4	Vertical Force

Figure 6. Force plate coordinate system.

2.2. Force Plate Data Acquisition

To acquire the GRF data during the gait analysis, the participant is always oriented to walk barefoot or wearing shoes, at him/her self selected speed, along the pathway covered by the experimental flooring and over one or two force platforms, embedded in the data collection room floor. As the participant step on the force platform, the force applied on it is detected by sensors and the electrical signals are amplified and recorded on a computer. It is important the participants be aware about the force plate locations so the gait performed is closer to normal gait pattern of the participant. Also, during data acquisition on the force platform, it is important to observe if the participant foot hits the force plate during the entire support phase. If it does not occur, this trial must be disregard because the data will be changed.

After the data acquisition to determine the optimal data filtering frequency the residual analysis is applied.

2.3. Residual Analysis

Residual analysis is used to determine the optimal theoretical cutoff frequency. For such, a noisy signal is filtered with various cutoff frequencies, close to the cutoff frequency accredited as the most appropriate. After, the root mean square error (mean residual) of each filtered signal is calculated. The residue of each filtered signal is then analyzed graphically taking into consideration the chosen cut off frequency. As shown in the figure below (Figure 7).

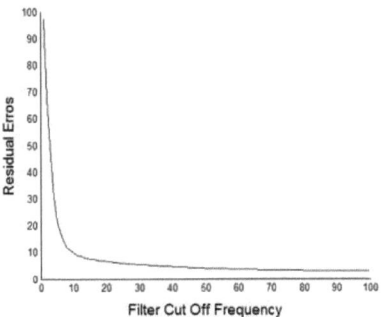

Figure 7. Residual Analysis.

According to Winter (1990), the projection between the residuals and the cutoff frequencies of the filter provides a profile of the curve with an abrupt increase at a given instant. This abrupt increase in the profile of the projection between residuals and the frequencies determines the cutoff frequency of the theoretical optimal filter cutoff. Also, the root mean square error is also calculated as a function of the signal, this analysis enables you to check which intensity of the filter.

2.4. Force Plate Data Normalization

In order to compare the data acquired by a force platform between different individuals and/or different conditions and repetitions, it is necessary to normalize the amplitude of these data (Figure 8a). The normalization can be performed by means of the value of the body weight of the subject, where the GRF data of an individual is divided by his/her body weight (Figure 8b).

It is also possible to normalize the temporal duration of the GRF. This is necessary to compare different trials and different subjects thanks to the variability of human locomotion. The temporal normalization stipulates that the beginning of the GRF data corresponds to 0% and the final to 100%, then the mathematical procedure called interpolation is used to generate a number of points between 0 and 100 for different repetitions (Figure 8c).

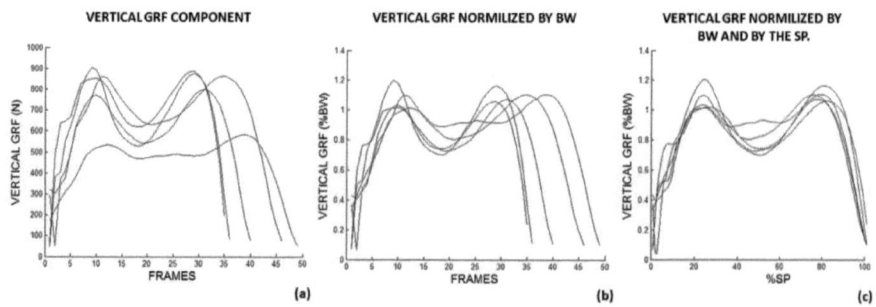

Figure 8. Ground reaction force data normalization.

20

2.5. The Ground Reaction Forces Components and the RCOF

The Fz ground reaction force has a greater magnitude than the other GRF components (anterior-posterior and lateral) characterized by two peaks and one valley. Generally, these peaks are of slightly higher magnitude than body weight. The first peak is observed during the first half of the support phase and features the absorption peak, which is when the foot absorbs body weight immediately after heel contact with the ground (Larish et al., 1988). The second peak is observed at the end of the support phase and it is known as the propulsion peak. It pushes against the ground to start the next step (Hamill & Knutzen, 2009). The valley between the two peaks is slightly smaller in magnitude than the body weight valley that occurs when the foot is in a flat position on the ground.

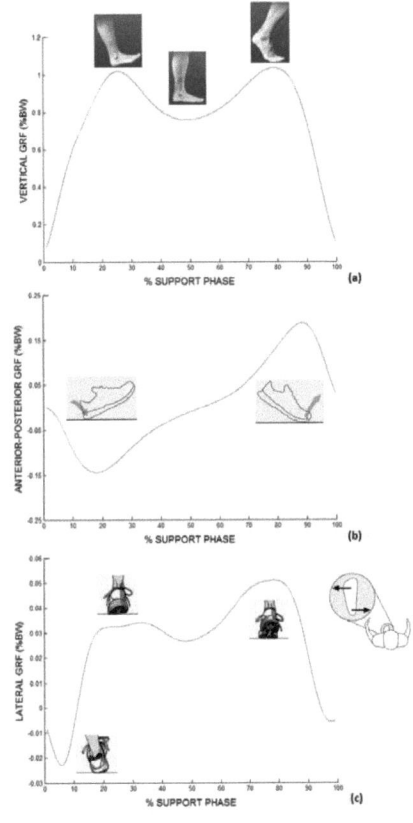

Figure 9. The ground reaction forces components.

The Fy GRF component has a negative phase (deceleration) during the first half of support and a positive phase (acceleration) during the other half of support. In the first half of the support phase, the foot pushes forward on the floor and, consequently, the GRF is directed backwards. In the second half of the support phase, the foot pushes the ground backwards and, consequently, the GRF is directed forward. Thus, the phase represents a negative rate of decrease for the body and the positive phase is accelerating the body forward (Winter, 1991). The peak strength for each of these phases

21

during walking is approximately equivalent to ~15% of the magnitude of body weight, and almost coincides in time with the two peaks of the vertical component of GRF (Larish et al., 1988).

The Fx GRF component has a very small magnitude (Whittle, 2007), and its variability component may be due to the diversity in foot positioning, which may be pointing inwards (adduction of the foot) or outwards (abduction of the foot) during the period of support.

After all the procedures described above, the instantaneous RCOF is calculated as the ratio of the shear force to the normal GRF during standing (Chang et al., 2012; Redfern et al., 2001) as described in Equation 3.

$$COF = \frac{\sqrt{(FY)^2 + (FX)^2}}{FZ} \tag{3}$$

Chapter 3. Effects of flooring on ground reaction forces and required coefficient of friction: elderly adult vs. middle-aged adult barefoot gait

In the previous Chapters the definition of COF and RCOF were presented. However, several gait parameters associated gait are noted for influencing friction demand characteristics. In the Chapter 3 the effect of flooring, age (middle-aged versus elderly adults) and gender in the RCOF during barefoot gait is discussed.

3.1. Introduction

Previous research has investigated the effects of age on the ability to walk on different flooring, e.g., carpet versus vinyl (Willmott, 1986; Dickinson et al., 2001). However, contradictory results were found depending on the gait velocity on these flooring types (Willmott, 1986; Dickinson et al., 2001). Changes in gait speed and step length during ambulation over two different surfaces such as carpet and vinyl flooring may influence the outcome of slips and falls, especially for the elderly. Understanding how older adults adapt to walking on different flooring types may provide useful information for the design of interventions to reduce falls in older people.

At the interface between the foot and the ground, footwear is likely to influence balance control and the risk of experiencing slips and trips while walking. The shoe type and sole material affect the available friction between the foot and the support surface. Because many falls occur when older adults walk barefoot inside their home or in a familiar environment (Menz et al., 2006), understanding their behavior while walking barefoot on different flooring should provide new insights about the risk of falls in the elderly population.

In general, elderly adults walk slower than young adults, with a higher heel contact velocity and a shorter step length (Lockhart, 1997; Lockhart et al., 2003; Burnfield and Powers, 2003; Kim and Lockhart, 2006; Menz et al., 2006; Seo and Kim, 2013). It has been suggested that these age-related gait adaptations influence the likelihood of slip-induced falls (Lockhart et al., 2003). Another factor that should be taken into account is gender differences. According to Lach (2005), gender is the most important covariant associated with the fear of falling. Women with balance and gait difficulty resulting in unsteadiness, multiple falls, and low self-rated health are at greatest risk (Lach, 2005).

Although fall risk factors among the elderly have been well studied (Lockhart, 1997; Lockhart et al., 2003; Burnfield and Powers, 2003; Kim and Lockhart, 2006; Menz et al., 2006; Seo and Kim, 2013), it could be interesting to understand the strategies adopted by middle-aged and elderly adults when walking over different flooring. We are interested in comparing older adults (60-70 years old) (O'Loughlin et al., 1994), whose risk of falling is relatively high, with a group of adults close in age (40-50 years old) with a lower risk of falling. Previous studies have only compared RCOF strategies in the elderly with control groups of young adults (20-30 years old) (Lockhart, 1997; Lockhart et al., 2003; Burnfield and Powers, 2003; Kim and Lockhart, 2006; Menz et al., 2006; Seo and Kim, 2013).

Therefore, the aim of this study was to investigate the effect of flooring on the RCOF during barefoot gait according to age (middle-aged versus elderly adults) and gender. Our goal was to test the following hypotheses: (a) differences in the RCOF variables can be found during barefoot gait on different flooring; (b) differences can be observed in the RCOF between elderly adults and middle-aged adults; and (c) gender differences in the RCOF can be observed during barefoot gait.

3.2. Methods

3.2.1. Participants

The Research Ethics Committee of the University of Campinas approved this study (UNICAMP protocol No. 319/2011), and the volunteers gave written informed consent to participate. Twenty healthy subjects volunteered in this study, and they were divided into two age groups: elderly adults (EA, n=10) and middle-aged adults (MA, n=10). Table 1 shows the anthropometric data for each group. The subjects recruited for this study were healthy (without known musculoskeletal, neurologic, cardiac, or pulmonary diagnoses), community dwelling, and ambulatory without an assistive device.

Table 1. Anthropometric data.

Group	N	Age (years)	Body Mass (kg)	Height (cm)
EA males	5	67.4±5.02	74.52±14.21	164.04±11.44
EA females	5	67.8±6.05	69.80±16.34	162.5±6.64
MA males	5	48.2±6.22	78.75±8.23	166.58±9.28
MA females	5	47.6±3.32	70.76±11.98	166.24±8.21
EA	10	67.6±5.25	72.17±14.66	166.41±8.26
MA	10	47.90±5.47	74.76±10.57	163.27±8.85
Males	10	57.7±11.92	70.28±13.52	164.37±7.3
Females	10	57.8±11.43	76.64±11.17	162.31±9.91

Legend: EA = Elderly Adult group; MA = Middle-aged Adult group; N = sample size.

3.2.2. Flooring Classification

Three flooring types under four experimental conditions were used to evaluate the study volunteers:

- *Homogeneous vinyl (HOV):* Homogeneous single-layer vinyl flooring (Pavifloor Prisma tile, 2 mm thickness, 2X8 m, ref. 909, charcoal, Tarkett Fademac);

- *Heterogeneous vinyl (HTV)*: Compact flexible vinyl floor covering (Chinese Teak natural, 2.50 mm thickness, 2X8 m, Imagine Wood, Tarkett Fademac);

- *Carpet:* Needle-punch carpet (plain quality needle-punch carpet, 100% pet fiber, 2 mm thickness, 2X8 m, Flortex Eco Inylbra);

- *Mixed:* To simulate a person walking from one room to another room with different flooring, a mixed condition was included. As illustrated in Figure 3d, the first 4 m of the pathway was covered by HTV, and the second 4 m of the pathway was covered by HOV.

To characterize the flooring used in this study, the static coefficient of friction (μ^s) was calculated using a pulley test. Figure 10a illustrates the test and the resulting μ^s. The chosen flooring was positioned on a force platform (Kistler 9286BA), and over this flooring a halter (H1) was positioned weighing 18.42 kg. Halter H1 was pulled by another halter (H2) weighing 17.32 kg. H1 was connected to H2 by a steel cable that slid on a system of three rollers, one fixed on the floor (R1) and two on the laboratory roof (R2 and R3). From the plot of the coefficient of friction of the force plate as a function of time, μ_e was determined as the maximum friction prior to the start of movement (Figure 10b). The μ_e values for all the flooring chosen for this study were approximately 0.5, which is within the standards of safety according to Templer (1992) and Miller (1983) (see Figures 10c, 10d, 10e and 10f).

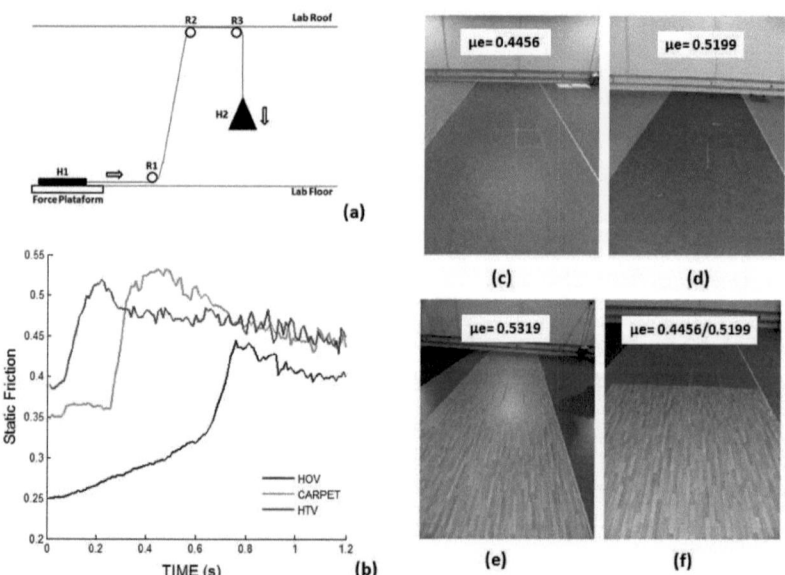

Figure 10. Illustration of the pulley test (a); illustration of the static friction curves (b), and, the flooring conditions with the pulley tests results: Homogeneous Vinyl (HOV - c); Carpet (d); Heterogeneous Vinyl (HTV – e); Mixed (HOV and HTV – f).

26

3.2.3. Experimental Procedures

The participant was asked to walk barefoot, at his or her selected speed, along a pathway of the experimental flooring material, beneath which two force platforms (Kistler 9286BA) were embedded in the data collection room floor, as shown in Figure 3. Possible effects of the participant's chosen speed on the results were tested, and no significant differences were found related to the flooring condition (p=0.710), age group (p=0.944) or gender (p=0.417). The participants were aware of the force plate locations. Three trials were performed for each experimental condition. Because of the difficulties associated with changing flooring conditions, all subjects accomplished the tasks in the same order: HOV, carpet, HTV and mixed.

The ground reaction force data were normalized by the subject's body weight (%BW) and expressed as a function of the percentage of the support phase. Data acquisition was performed using BioWare software (Version 4.0.x). Kinetic raw data were filtered using a 2nd order low-pass digital Butterworth filter with a cut-off frequency of 10 Hz. The filtering data parameters were chosen after a Residual Analysis. An algorithm developed in Matlab was used to filter the raw data and to calculate the dependent variables.

The independent variables were the type of surface (HOV, HTV, carpet or mixed), age group (EA or MA) and gender (female or male). The discrete variables used in the study were as follows:

RCOF1: the local maximum of the instantaneous COF curve occurring at ~20% of the duration of the stance phase of the gait in the weight acceptance (see Figure 11);

RCOF2: the instantaneous COF peak at ~90% of the duration of the stance phase of gait in the push off (see Figure 11).

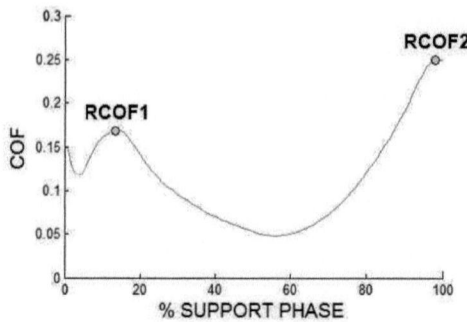

Figure 11. Illustration of the RCOF curve represented by the average curve over all healthy females participants in the HOV condition.

3.2.4. Statistical Analysis

A two-sample t-test was performed to compare the anthropometric variables (height and weight) between age groups. A linear mixed-effects model (West et al., 2007) for repeated measures was performed to analyze the possible effects of flooring, age and gender on the dependent friction variables. The repeated covariance type chosen for the mixed linear model was scaled identity. Three trials for each flooring condition were considered in the statistical procedures. The model applied used three main factors. The first analysis factor was the flooring, which was treated as a repeated measures factor with four sublevels (HOV, carpet, HTV and mixed). The second factor analyzed was age, with two sublevels (EA and MA). The third factor was gender (male and female). The first effect was considered as a within-subjects factor, and the second and third effects were considered as between-subjects factors. The Bonferroni test of pairwise comparisons was computed for every level of combination of factors and interactions. SPSS software (SPSS for Windows, version 19.0) was used for the statistical analysis, with a level of significance of $\alpha \leq 0.05$ for all tests.

The partial eta squared ($\eta^2_{partial}$) value was calculated as in Equation 4 to verify the practical relevance of the main effects and interactions. As proposed by Richardson (2011), in this study, partial η^2 values >0.01 were categorized as low, >0.06 as medium, and >0.14 as high.

28

$$\eta_{partial}^2 = \left(\frac{\text{Full model residual variance}}{\text{Full model residual variance} + \text{Reduced model residual variance}} \right) \qquad (4)$$

3.3. Results

The two-sample t-test revealed no significant differences between the EA and MA groups for body mass ($F_{1,19}$=0.206; p=0.655) and height ($F_{1,19}$=0.007; p=0.936).

The mixed model analysis revealed significant differences for the three main factors (flooring, age and gender), with no interaction between them. When the flooring types were compared during the loading response phase, the participants demonstrated a greater RCOF1 on carpet than on the HOV or HTV flooring ($F_{3,480}$=3.273; p=0.021; $\eta_{partial}^2$=0.68; Figure 12a). The $\eta_{partial}^2$ value shows that the relevance of this effect was high.

In the push-off phase, the RCOF2 was statistically greater when the subjects walked on carpet than when they walked on the HOV flooring, with a medium level of practical relevance for this main factor ($F_{3,480}$=4.182; p=0.006; $\eta_{partial}^2$=0.11; Figure 12b).

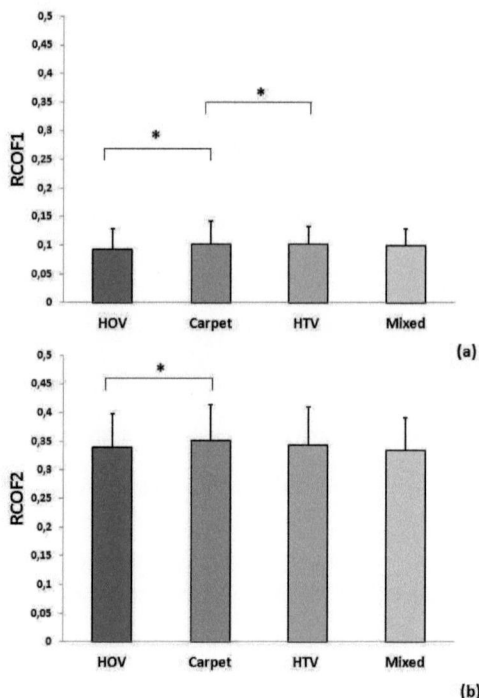

(a)

(b)

Figure 12. Required coefficient of friction at loading response (RCOF1) and push-off (RCOF2) phases of gait. Values expressed in terms of means and standard deviation. Legend: * = p<0.05.

The EA group had statistically smaller RCOF2 values than the MA group, with a high practical relevance for the factor ($F_{1,480}$=42.948; p=0.0001; $\eta^2_{partial}$=0.61; Figure 13a). Moreover, when gender effects were compared, the male subjects had a lower RCOF1 than the female subjects, with a medium level of practical relevance ($F_{1,480}$=7.979; p=0.005; $\eta^2_{partial}$=0.04; Figure 13b).

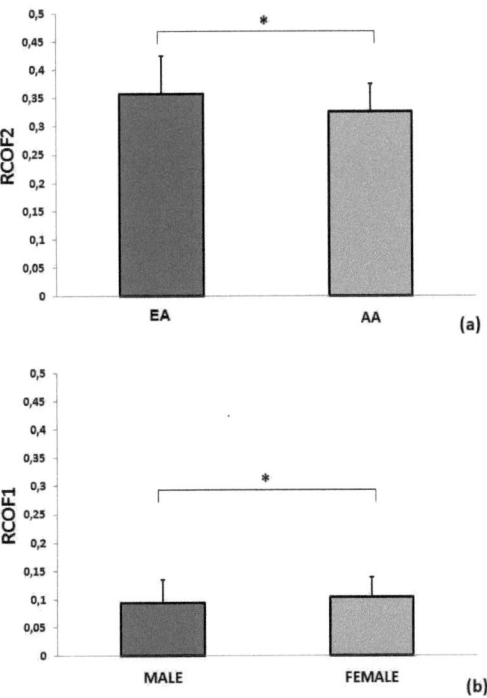

Figure 13. Means and Standard deviations and statistical results for Age (a) and gender (b) effects. Legend: * = p=0.001.

3.5. Discussion

This research project was undertaken to provide a better understanding of how flooring, age and gender influence foot-floor friction in the gait of healthy middle-aged and elderly male and female subjects. Barefoot gait was selected for analysis because according to Menz et al. (2006), a higher risk of falling indoors is associated with going barefoot. The required coefficient of friction at the loading response and push-off phases of gait were used as experimental variables because it is well known in the literature that these variables are related to the risk of a fall and also make it possible to mechanically characterize the foot-floor interaction.

The main result obtained in the present study was that the three main factors tested in the statistical model (flooring, age and gender) were significant and had practical relevance ranging from medium to high. No interaction was found among flooring, age and gender; therefore, no conclusion was possible regarding distinctive behaviors of the EA or MA groups, or of the male or female participants, with each flooring type.

The RCOF was higher during barefoot gait on carpet than on vinyl flooring (HTV and HOV) in the deceleration phase of gait (i.e., the loading response) as well as in the push-off phase (i.e., the terminal stance), confirming the first hypothesis of the present study and suggesting that carpet is the safest flooring of the three types analyzed in the present study.

It is well known that surface roughness plays an important role in floor slipperiness when subjects wear walking shoes (Kim et al., 2013; Kim and Nagata, 2008; Chang et al., 2012; Lockhart et al., 2003). Our results confirm this finding in barefoot walking.

The effect of the flooring condition on the friction variables was not surprising; however, it demonstrates that this aspect should be considered during gait analyses and gait investigations. Because friction is a relevant factor in gait patterns, the proper description and control of this variable are important for experimental design in gait analysis. However, because these variables are related to age and gender, they could be used alone or in correlation in further studies.

The study found different RCOF behavior in the EA and MA subjects. This could be due to plantar sensitivity. Plantar sensitivity is an important source of information for balance control because it codifies the changes in pressure under the feet, especially during gait. This information reaches the brain, which senses the body position and, if necessary, generates postural reflexes to maintain an upright position and dynamic balance during gait (Kavounoudias et al., 1998; Wang and Lin, 2008).

Compared to the barefoot condition, walking shoes could potentially interfere with the detection of plantar surface stimulation. Such interference might be inconsequential for individuals with intact plantar sensitivity. However, EA often have reduced plantar sensitivity (Perry, 2006).

A further reduction in plantar sensory feedback while walking barefoot might lead to insufficient afferent input for locomotion control in EA and MA, and consequently, a cautious gait

32

might need to be adopted. Further studies are needed to determine the relationship between barefoot gait plantar sensitivity and the effect of more challenging flooring on gait. A false subjective perception of slipperiness might lead to an inappropriate gait pattern, which might result in a higher probability of a slip-induced fall in the elderly population.

The results of the present study are in agreement with previous studies that have shown that the peak RCOF varies with age (Lockhart, 1997) and gender (Burnfield and Powers, 2003).

When the age groups were compared, the EA group had a lower RCOF during the toe-off phase. This adaptation is thought to result in more stable or safer gait patterns in the elderly. Future studies exploring this developmental effect could attempt to determine the exact time at which the risk of falls becomes pronounced in this population and could also investigate the possibility of effective interventions to reduce falls in the elderly population.

There were also gender differences in the RCOF. Female participants had higher RCOF values during heel contact. This was also observed by Li et al. (2001) and Chao et al. (1983), who found that women exhibited greater vertical GRF than men. Burnfield and Powers (2003) found that the peak RCOF varied with gender; females generated higher peak RCOF values than males at a slow walking speed, whereas males generated higher peak RCOF values than females at a fast walking speed. The structural differences in the female hip and knee may result in differences in their movement patterns (Mizuno et al., 2001; Ferber et al., 2003). This suggests that some intrinsic characteristics, such as skeletal alignment, muscle strength and anthropometric parameters, may contribute to gender and age differences in gait performance.

3.6. Conclusion

In conclusion, friction during barefoot gait was found to be affected by flooring type, gender and age. Carpet was the safest flooring in terms of the required coefficient of friction. When elderly adults were compared to middle-aged adults, they demonstrated a reduced required coefficient of friction during the toe-off phase, and gender differences were observed in the RCOF during the heel contact phase in barefoot gait.

Much of the research on falls has focused on how the aging process affects gait. The problem with this clinical focus is that little thought has been given to the environment, such as flooring differences in the patient's home. The fact that EA are particularly challenged under these circumstances could be exploited in designing rehabilitation exercises to improve functional mobility and reduce falls with advanced age; in particular, the role of patients' plantar sensitivity during barefoot gait could be explored. In fact, a reduced incidence of falling in EA has been demonstrated following an exercise intervention using an obstacle course designed with different flooring conditions and obstacles to foot placement.

Chapter 4. Effects of flooring and hemibody on ground reaction forces and coefficient of friction in stroke gait

The study presented in Chapter 3 elucidate that the RCOF in healthy elderly adults in barefoot

gait varies according the flooring type, the age and the gender. But does the flooring type have the

same effect in pathological gait? This Chapter answer this question exploring the effect of flooring in

the GRF and RCOF in stroke gait.

4.1. Introduction

Previous studies investigated the RCOF in pathological groups (Buczek et al., 1990; Burnfield

et al., 2003; Durá et al., 2005; Haynes and Lockhart, 2012). Buczek et al. (1990) found that persons

with a disability (amputations, broken leg, osteotomy of the fifth metatarsal) had higher peak RCOF

during level walking when compared to persons without a disability. Durá et al. (2005) also examined

a diverse sample including amputees, Parkinson's disease, and stroke individuals. Their results

suggested that the RCOF for all subjects other than amputees was similar to that for normal walkers,

while that for the amputees was substantially higher (approximately 0.25 versus 0.39). Burnfield et

al. (2003) conducted a study to examine the difference in RCOF among young, healthy elderly, and

elderly subjects with diabetes mellitus, lower extremity arthritis and unilateral stroke. No significant

differences were found between any of these groups, in agreement with Durá et al. (2005). The lack

of significant differences in RCOF among subject groups suggested that individuals with the selected

medical conditions were at no greater risk of slipping when walking at a self-selected step than were

healthy older or younger adults.

Examination of the collective results of these studies (Buczek et al., 1990; Burnfield et al.,

2003; Durá et al., 2005), suggests that only one class of individuals with walking impairments (i.e., those with prosthetics/amputations) is likely to require higher levels of RCOF than do normal walkers. Moreover, these studies (Buczek et al., 1990; Burnfield et al., 2003; Durá et al., 2005) did not systematically examine a unique medical condition (i.e., stroke); different medical conditions analyzed at the same time can have higher data variability and enshroud some results.

With regards of these results (Buczek et al., 1990; Burnfield et al., 2003; Durá et al., 2005; Haynes and Lockhart, 2012) should be interesting to explore the stroke walking over different flooring and this factor influence in the GRF and RCOF.

Studies suggested asymmetrical spatial-temporal, kinematic (Sadeghi et al., 2000) and RCOF (Seo and Kim 2013a, 2013b) differences between dominant legs and non-dominant legs in healthy young adults, most of the studies found no difference in leg strength between legs unless a young individual had experienced unilateral leg injury (Holder-Powell and Rutherford, 2000). However, significant strength or power imbalance was presented in the elderly fallers in comparison to the non-fallers (Skelton, 2002).

Moreover, in pathological gait marked asymmetry has been noted between the stroke subjects' affected and less affected lower limbs. Decreased GRF have been reported on the affected limb relative to the less affected limb in the gait of persons with stroke (Titianova and Tarkka, 1995; Morita et al., 1995).

As shown, stroke gait analysis has increased in the last years, however, the possible effect of flooring in association with stroke hemibodies, on gait parameters such as ground reaction forces and friction, to the best of our knowledge, has not yet been studied. So, the aim of this study was to investigate the effect of flooring in the GRF and foot/floor friction during stroke gait considering this population's lowers limb asymmetry (affected and less affected lower limbs). It was hypothesized that: the stroke group will exhibit lower RCOF than the healthy age-matched peers, especially when the different flooring types are compared.

4.2. Methods

4.2.1. Participants

The Research Ethics Committee approved this study (protocol No. 319/2011) and the volunteers gave written informed consent to participate.

The hemiparetic group (HG) consisted of 12 individuals affected by stroke and the control group (CG) consisted of 12 healthy adults. The Table 2 describes the anthropometric data for each group.

Table 2. Anthropometric data.

VARIABLES	HG	CG
N	12 (5 females and 7 males)	12 (5 females and 7 males)
Age (years)	62.83 ± 6.86	63.58 ± 6.94
Body Mass (kg)	69.50 ± 13.96	73.08 ± 14.31
Height (m)	1.68 ± 0.06	1.69 ± 0.05
TAS (months)	6.1 ± 2.8	-
Fugl-Meyer	88.25 ± 6.95	-
Berg Balance Scale	47.16 ± 8.13	-
DGI	16.25±4.13	-
Mini-mental	21.33±4.61	-

Legend: N = number of participants; TAS = time after stroke; DGI = Dynamic Gait Index Scale; HG = hemiplegic group; CG = control group.

4.2.2. Experimental Procedures

The experimental procedures of this study were the same presented in Chapter 3 pages 39 to 41.

The independent variables were: type of flooring surface (HOV, HTV, carpet and mixed) and hemibody (the hemibody of stroke patients were classified as affected (AS) or less affected (LAS) and the control group left limb (CG).

The variables used in the study were obtained from the GRF components curve and the coefficient of friction (COF):

(a) **Fz GRF component:** first peak of impact (Fz1), maximum value of first curve peak; valley (Fz2), minimum value between the first and the second peak of the vertical component curve; and the propulsion peak (Fz3), maximum value of the second curve peak (Figure 14a).

(b) **Fy GRF component:** negative phase (deceleration or braking - Fy1), minimum value of the anterior-posterior GRF in the first half of the support phase and positive phase (acceleration - Fy2), maximum value of the anterior-posterior GRF in the second half of the support phase (Figure 14b).

(c) **Fx GRF component :** maximum lateral force (Fx1), minimum value of the curve; first maximum medial force (Fx2), maximum value of the curve on in the first half of the support phase; and second maximum medial force (Fx3), maximum value of the curve in the second half of the support phase (Figure 14c).

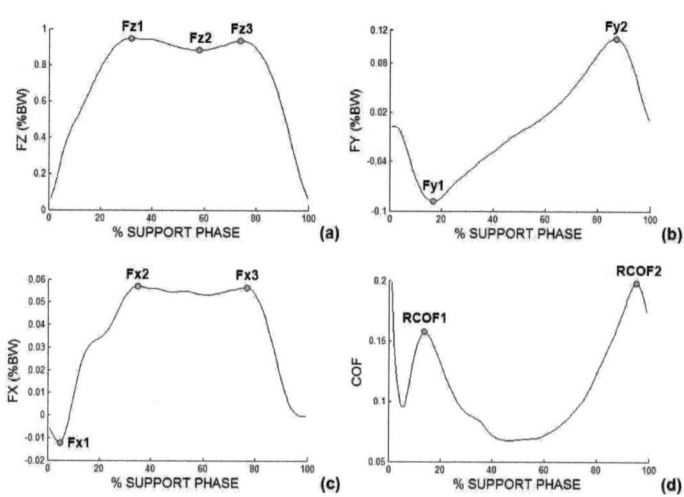

Figure 14. Illustration of the GRF component curves represented by the average curve for all stroke participants in the HOV condition and the discrete variables of the: (a) FZ - GRF vertical component; (b) FY - GRF anterior-posterior component; (c) FX - GRF lateral component; (d) COF – coefficient of friction. Legend: %BW: percentage of body weight.

(d) **The RCOF1 and RCOF2:** to determine these variables, the same procedures presented in Chapter 3 were apply here (Figure 14d).

(e) **Contact time:** defined as the time elapsed between heel strike and toe off and it is expressed in seconds.

4.2.3. Statistical Analysis

For the statistical analysis, firstly the differences between right and left lower limbs for CG were tested. The Kolmoronov-Smirnov Test revealed non-normal distribution therefore Mann-Whitney Test ($\alpha \leq 0.05$) was applied. Since no statistical difference was found between limbs the left one was selected to represent the control group hemibody for all comparisons.

The comparisons among flooring type (HOV, carpet, HTV and Mixed) for each hemibody (affected, unaffected and control) were performed by the Friedman test for related samples. Also, the comparisons among hemibodies (AS, LAS and CG) for each flooring type (HOV, carpet, HTV and Mixed) were performed by the Kruskall-Wallis test for independent samples. Bonferroni pair-wise comparisons were computed for all-level of combination of factors and interactions. All differences in effect were analyzed in the SPSS ® software (SPSS for Windows, version 19.0) with a significant level $\alpha \leq 0.05$ for all tests.

4.3. Results

The ANOVA one way test revealed no significant differences between stroke and control groups for age ($F_{1,23}=0.071$; $p=0.793$), body mass ($F_{1,23}=0.385$; $p=0.541$) and height ($F_{1,23}=0.352$; $p=0.559$).

There was difference regarding the flooring surface for the AS for the following variables: Fy1, Fy2 and RCOF2. The AS performed lower breaking, acceleration and RCOF2 during the walking on HOV in comparison to the other flooring. The Table 3 presents the statistical test results for the comparisons between AS and flooring conditions.

The same behavior was assumed by the LAS in the acceleration phase. Moreover, the LAS presented different behavior in RCOF2 for each flooring. The HOV and mixed presented lower RCOF2 than the other surfaces (see Table 4). However, there were no differences among surfaces and the ground reaction forces and RCOF variables for the control group.

The Kruskall-Wallis test revealed differences among hemibodies and flooring type for: Fx2, Fy1, Fy2, Fz2; Fz3 and contact time. For these variables, in all the flooring conditions the stroke AS and LAS did not present differences, but differences were found between the stroke group with the control group. However, for the Fx2 there are no differences between hemibodies in the HOV. The Table 4 presents these comparisons among lower limbs (AS, LAS and CG) for each flooring type (HOV, carpet, HTV and Mixed). Moreover, for the RCOF1 and RCOF2 in the HOV, Carpet, HTV and Mixed conditions the stroke AS and LAS performed lower dynamic friction during the hell contact than CG (Table 4). Also the stroke AS performed lower RCOF during the push off phase than the stroke LAS and CG (Table 4).

Table 3. Friedman test results: comparisons among flooring type (HOV, carpet, HTV and Mixed) for each lower limb (affected and less affected) for each variable presented in means and standard deviations.

VAR	AFFECTED SIDE				X²	P	LESS AFFECTED SIDE				X²	P
	HOV	Carpet	HTV	Mixed			HOV	Carpet	HTV	Mixed		
Fx1(%BW)	-.02±0.01	-.02±0.01	-.02±0.02	-.02±0.01	1.941	0.585	-.022±0.01	-.026±0.02	-.025±0.02	-.024±0.02	2.094	0.553
Fx2(%BW)	0.05±0.01	0.06±0.01	0.058±0.01	0.06±0.016	1.309	0.727	0.06±0.03	0.06±0.02	0.06±0.02	0.06±0.02	1.111	0.774
Fx3(%BW)	0.06±0.01	0.06±0.02	0.06±0.02	0.06±0.018	0.266	0.966	0.06±0.03	0.06±0.03	0.06±0.03	0.06±0.02	1.413	0.703
Fy1(%BW)	-.10±0.05°•	-.12±0.05°	-.12±0.05•	-.11±0.061	8.378	**0.039**	-.104±0.04	-.118±0.05	-.111±0.04	-.120±0.04	6.936	0.074
Fy2(%BW)	**0.11±0.06°•+**	**0.12±0.06°**	**0.13±0.06•**	**0.13±0.058+**	**14.179**	**0.003**	**0.12±0.06°•+**	**0.14±0.06°**	**0.14±0.06•**	**0.14±0.06+**	**19.291**	**0.001**
Fz1(%BW)	1.00±0.09	1.05±0.09	1.03±0.09	1.02±0.07	5.431	0.143	1.00±0.07	1.03±0.08	1.01±0.07	1.02±0.07	3.519	0.318
Fz2(%BW)	0.86±0.05	0.86±0.07	0.85±0.07	0.85±0.053	2.024	0.567	0.88±0.06	0.86±0.06	0.87±0.06	0.87±0.06	4.853	0.183
Fz3(%BW)	1.00±0.05	1.01±0.06	1.01±0.06	1.01±0.07	3.543	0.315	1.01±0.07	1.02±0.06	1.01±0.07	1.02±0.08	1.292	0.731
RCOF1	0.17±0.03	0.18±0.03	0.17±0.03	0.16±0.05	2.911	0.406	0.16±0.04	0.17±0.03	0.17±0.03	0.17±0.04	4.911	0.178
RCOF2	**0.23±0.07°•+**	**0.28±0.1°**	**0.28±0.1•**	**0.25±0.07+**	**9.264**	**0.026**	**0.28±0.07°•***	**0.31±0.08°∞**	**0.33±0.1^**	**0.26±0.09∞Δ**	**18.633**	**0.0001**
CT(s)	0.96±1.13	0.93±1.13	0.70±0.18	0.71±0.13	4.453	0.217	0.86±0.24	1±1.22	0.79±0.18	0.77±0.14	6.887	0.076

Legend: VAR = variables; %BW = normalized by body weight; CT = contact time; X² = Friedman test values; P = p-values; ° = differences between HOV and Carpet; • = differences between HOV and HTV; + = differences between HOV and Mixed; ∞ = differences between Carpet and Mixed; Δ = differences between HTV and Mixed.

41

Table 4. Kruskall-Wallis test results: comparisons among lower limbs (AS, LAS and CG) for each flooring type (HOV, carpet, HTV and Mixed) each variable presented in means and standard deviations.

VAR	HOV			H2	P	CARPET			H2	P
	AS	LAS	CG			AS	LAS	CG		
Fx1(%BW)	-.02±0.01	-.02±0.01	-.02±0.01	0.413	0.813	-.023±0.01	-.026±0.02	-.021±0.01	0.451	0.798
Fx2(%BW)	0.05±0.01	0.06±0.03	0.05±0.02	4.964	0.084	0.06±0.01*	0.06±0.02°	0.04±0.01*°	9.234	0.01
Fx3(%BW)	0.06±0.01	0.06±0.03	0.05±0.02	0.154	0.926	0.06±0.02	0.06±0.03	0.05±0.01	1.562	0.458
Fy1(%BW)	-.11±0.05*	-.10±0.04°	0.15±0.04*°	20.458	0.0001	-.12±0.05*	-.12±0.05°	-.16±0.04*°	12.774	0.0002
Fy2(%BW)	0.11±0.06*	0.12±0.06°	0.18±0.03*°	25.760	0.0001	0.12±0.06*	0.14±0.06°	0.20±0.03*°	26.381	0.0001
Fz1(%BW)	1.00±0.09	1.00±0.07	1.04±0.17	5.852	0.054	1.05±0.09	1.03±0.08	1.04±0.17	2.698	0.259
Fz2(%BW)	0.86±0.05*	0.88±0.06°	0.74±0.12*°	37.531	0.0001	0.86±0.07*	0.86±0.06°	0.75±0.11*°	26.930	0.0001
Fz3(%BW)	1.00±0.06*	1.01±0.07°	1.06±0.13*°	22.875	0.0001	1.01±0.06*	1.02±0.06°	1.06±0.13*°	19.244	0.0001
RCOF1	0.17±0.03*	0.16±0.03°	0.09±0.03*°	40.067	0.0001	0.18±0.03*	0.17±0.03°	0.09±0.04*°	43.051	0.0001
RCOF2	0.23±0.07*Δ	0.28±0.07°Δ	0.32±0.04*°	21.007	0.0001	0.28±0.1*Δ	0.31±0.08°Δ	0.33±0.04*°	33.700	0.0001
CT (s)	0.96±1.13*	0.86±0.24°	0.63±0.08*°	25.131	0.0001	0.93±1.13*	1±1.22°	0.64±0.06*°	13.367	0.0001

VAR	HTV			H2	P	MIXED			H2	P
	AS	LAS	CG			AS	LAS	CG		
Fx1 (%BW)	-.023±0.01	-.025±0.02	-.021±0.01	0.319	0.853	-.022±0.01	-.024±0.02	-.02±0.01	0.930	0.628
Fx2 (%BW)	0.06±0.01*	0.06±0.02°	0.04±0.01*°	10.617	0.005	0.06±0.01*	0.06±0.02°	0.04±0.01*°	16.441	0.0001
Fx3 (%BW)	0.06±0.02	0.06±0.03	0.05±0.01	1.867	0.393	0.06±0.01	0.06±0.03	0.05±0.01	2.824	0.244
Fy1 (%BW)	-.12±0.05*	-.11±0.04°	-.14±0.04*°	8.155	0.017	-.11±0.06*	-.12±0.04°	-.15±0.04*°	10.551	0.005
Fy2 (%BW)	0.13±0.06*	0.14±0.06°	0.2±0.03*°	20.473	0.0001	0.13±0.05*	0.13±0.06°	0.19±0.03*°	23.012	0.0001
Fz1 (%BW)	1.03±0.09	1.01±0.07	1.04±0.17	4.126	0.127	1.02±0.07	1.02±0.07	1.04±0.17	3.241	0.198
Fz2 (%BW)	0.85±0.07*	0.87±0.06°	0.76±0.11*°	21.710	0.0001	0.85±0.05*	0.87±0.06°	0.76±0.12*°	25.598	0.0001
Fz3 (%BW)	1.01±0.06*	1.01±0.07°	1.06±0.12*°	23.928	0.0001	1.01±0.08*	1.02±0.08°	1.06±0.12*°	17.261	0.0001
RCOF1	0.18±0.03*	0.18±0.03°	0.10±0.04*°	40.067	0.0001	0.16±0.05*	0.17±0.04°	0.10±0.04*°	31.593	0.0001
RCOF2	0.28±0.1*Δ	0.32±0.1Δ	0.33±0.04*	29.661	0.0001	0.25±0.07*	0.26±0.09°	0.32±0.04*°	9.363	0.0009
CT(s)	0.70±0.18*	0.79±0.18°	0.65±0.08*°	9.261	0.01	0.71±0.13*	0.77±0.14°	0.64±0.06*°	16.389	0.0001

Legend: VAR = variables; %BW = normilized by body weight; CT = contact time; X^2 = Friedman test values; P = p-values; * = differences between AS and CG; ° = differences between LAS and CG; Δ = differences between AS and LAS.

4.4. Discussion

This study compared the gait of stroke patients to that of healthy age matched peers in an effort to quantify differences that may be predisposing the stroke population to falls in everyday environments.

When the hemibody effects were compared both AS and LAS for stroke group performed higher valley (Fz2) and lower propulsion peak (Fz3) than the CG, stroke patients may lose the heel-strike and push-off mechanism, altering the GRF pattern from 'M' to pathological shapes. These results are related to the stroke gait features, specially the main alterations found in the affected lower limb joints as decreased ankle, knee and hip flexion/extension range of motion (Carmo et al., 2012).

The lost of the heel-strike and push-off mechanism during stroke gait also contributed for the anterior-posterior (Fy) and lateral (Fx) ground reaction force components. The stroke AS and LAS performed higher braking (Fy1) and lower forward propulsion (Fy2) when compared with the CG for the anterior-postior forces. At the lateral components, the stroke LAS medial maximum force (Fx2) showed higher values than the AS and control group. This is reflected by a hemiplegic gait with reduced knee flexion at toe-off and mid-swing in the paretic limb (Chen et al., 2005).

Not only the dynamic friction but also the first peak (Fz1) and the negative peak (Fy1) in shear force are considered to be the most critical with respect to slips resulting in falls (Redfern et al., 2001). The results of this study showed that stroke patients have lower breaking and acceleration ability respectively during the heel strike and the toe off. Thus, for this population, the forces specially occurring at toe off are of critical importance in determining if the frictional capabilities of the foot/floor interface will be sufficient to prevent slips, and it also could be another relational aspect with increased falls occurrence of this population.

Contradicting Durá et al. (2005) and Burnfield et al. (2003), differences in hemibody for dynamic friction during the push off phase were also observed in this study. The control group presented higher dynamic friction than the stroke LAS and AS, and the LAS showed higher friction than the AS. Since the shear forces are higher near the heel contact and toe off phases (Redfern et al., 2001; Redfern and Dipasquale, 1998) these are the moments where slips occur more often. The toe off causes backward slip on the sole forepart, which can be more easily counteracted by stepping forward with the leading foot during normal gait (Grönqvist et al., 1999). As a results of the lack of ankle range of motion the stroke patients don't have the ability to easily counteracted the fall with this strategy.

Moreover, there were differences regarding the flooring surface for the stroke AS and LAS for RCOF2. It is well known that surface roughness plays an important role in floor slipperiness in walking shoes (Kim et al., 2013; Kim and Nagata, 2008; Lockhart et al., 2003). Our results confirm the same effect during the barefoot walking, more specifically when pathology is considered. It seems that even when stroke patients have loss of plantar proprioception (Lin et al., 2012) they are still able to detect the flooring roughness. However, false subjective perception of slipperiness might lead to an inappropriate gait pattern, which might result in higher probability of a slip-induced fall accident on the stroke population. So, understanding the relationship between the stroke gait parameters and friction demand characteristics may help identify slip prone individuals thereby reducing fall accidents.

Future studies should considerer the inclusion of spatiotemporal and kinematic variables such as the heel contact velocity and the acceleration of the whole body center-of-mass to analyze the stroke gait over different flooring. These variables could indicate further increase risk of slipping, for example, higher heel contact velocity can increase horizontal ground reaction force in relation to vertical ground reaction force and as a result, friction demand could increase. Furthermore, slower transitory acceleration of the whole body COM among the stroke can also increase friction demand at the foot/floor interface and increase risk of slipping.

4.5. Conclusion

This is the first study to report the relationship between hemibodies in dynamic friction variables of gait in persons after stroke during the walking on different flooring. The flooring effect was found on RCOF during the toe off for the AS and LAS. Therefore, the better understanding of the biomechanical differences between people with stroke and their healthy peers presented in the present paper revealed to be an important step to identify potential risk factors of slip injuries. In case of eliciting gait adjustments (during slip avoidance), stroke individuals' gait adaptation may encumber optimal gait adjustment strategy.

Chapter 5. The coefficient of friction alterations in stroke gait.

As we have been exploring in the previous Chapters of this thesis, the RCOF is represented by 2 instants in the loading response and toe off phases. Since in Chapter 4 we found differences in Stroke and control groups, could we also find differences in the RCOF curve shape when these two groups are compared? Also, could the RCOF curve of stroke patients a characteristic pattern? Also, in Chapter 4 the gait velocity seems to influence the presented results. So in this Chapter, to exclude the influence of walking velocity the RCOF variables are normalized by this parameter.

5.1. Introduction

Abnormal gait significantly limits the stroke patients' autonomy and capacity of participation, and also contributes to decrease their life quality (Wyller and Kirkevold 1999; Perry et al., 1995). Hemiplegia is one of the most common impairments observed after stroke and it contributes significantly to reduce gait performance. About 50% to 60% of patients that complete the standard rehabilitation after a stroke still experience some degree of motor impairment, and approximately 50% are at least partly dependent in activities-of-daily-living (Mayo et al., 1991). Thus, one of the earliest concerns of stroke patients and their families relates to walking issues (Mayo et al., 1991), therefore one of the focuses on the intervention after strokes is to treat gait abnormalities (Mayo et al., 1991).

The gait pattern of individuals post-stroke is often characterized by movement initiation delays, inefficient movement patterns on the hemiparetic side, decreased stance time on the paretic side, and premature toe off during terminal stance, when compared to healthy adults (Olney et al., 1991; Winter, 1983a, 1983b). Studies have shown that cognitive deficits, functional impairment, and impaired balance are related to fall incidence in stroke patients (Teasell and Kalra, 2004; Harris et al., 2005).

To the best of our knowledge, the COF curves during the gait of stroke patients have not yet been fully studied. So, our aim is to analyze the COF instantaneous curves of these patients during the barefoot gait and consequently kinetics aspects of hemiplegic gait.

5.2. Methods

5.2.1. Participants

The participants of this study as well the experimental procedures for motion analysis were the same as the one presented in Chapter 4. However, the data used for the comparisons between the stroke group and the aged matched control group were the data collected just in HOV condition.

5.2.2. Variables and Statistical Analysis

The COF curve was calculated as described in Equation 1, see this equation in Chapter 1. Then, as illustrated in Figure 15, the following parameters of the COF curves were calculated:

(a) RCOF1 (P_1): was calculated as the maximum value between the 9-15% of the COF curve;

(b) Valley1 (V_1): was calculated as the minimum value between the 15-80% of the COF curve;

(c) RCOF2 (P_2): was calculated as the maximum value between the 81-100% of the COF curve.

46

Since the COF can be affected by walking velocity, these variables were also normalized by the walking velocity (stride length/stride duration).

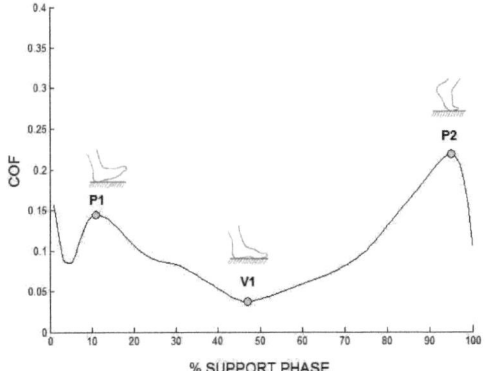

Figure 15. Illustration of COF curve variables. Legend: COF: coefficient of friction; %SUPPORT PHASE: percent of support phase; P_1 = $RCOF_1$; V_1 = $Valley_1$; P_2 = $RCOF_2$.

5.2.3. Statistical Analysis

In order to calculate the statistical analysis, the data normality was tested by Kolmoronov-Smirnov test. Then, to compare the differences between stroke hemibody (affected side - AS and less affected side - LAS) and control group, the parametric data was analyzed by one-way ANOVA and the Tukey post-hoc test ($\alpha \leq 0.05$); the nonparametric data was analyzed by Kruskall-Wallis test and the Bonferroni post-hoc test ($\alpha \leq 0.05$). Also, comparisons between the AS, LAS and CG COF instantaneous curves were made by the two sample T-test ($\alpha \leq 0.05$) comparing every 1% of gait cycle. The software SPSS (version 19) was used to perform all statistical analysis.

5.3. Results

The ANOVA one-way test have revealed no significant differences between stroke and control groups when considering age ($F_{1,23}=0.071$; $p=0.793$), body mass ($F_{1,23}=0.385$; $p=0.541$) and height ($F_{1,23}=0.352$; $p=0.559$).

Table 5 presents the discrete variable means and standard deviation for each group as well as the statistical results. When the COF curves' peaks and valleys were compared, differences were found in V_1nor, to which during the mid-stance phase both stroke AS and LAS presented higher values than the matched control group. Differences were also observed in P_2nor, during the terminal stance the control group presented lower values than the stroke AS and LAS.

Table 5.The discrete COF variables mean and standard deviation for each group and variable and the statistical results.

Variables	Groups			Statistics	P
	AS	LAS	Control		
P_1nor	0,25±0,08	0,28±0,15	0,17±0,03	KW=1,083	0,582
V_1nor	**0,09±0,06**•	**0,11±0,13**°	**0,03±0,01**•°	**KW=7,407**	**0,025**
P_2nor	**0,46±0,34**•	**0,40±0,18**°	**0,29±0,03**•°	**KW=8,722**	**0,013**

Legend: V_1nor = Valley1 normalized by the gait velocity; V_2nor = Valley2 normalized by the gait velocity; P_1nor = RCOF1 normalized by the gait velocity; P_2nor = RCOF2 normalized by the gait velocity; AS = stroke group affected side; LAS = stroke group less affected side; Control = Control group; • = differences between AS and Control; ° = differences between NAS and Control.

The COF instantaneous curves' analysis highlights the phases during the support phase where the Stroke patients AS and LAS have presented alterations compared to the control group, and it have shown differences in between the stroke symmetry (AS versus LAS).

When comparing AS and the control group (Figure 16a), differences were seen on initial contact (5% to 8% of the support phase), loading response (13% to 29% of the support phase), mid stance (46% to 67% of the support phase) and terminal stance to pre swing phases (77% to 70% of the support phase). When the LAS and the control group (Figure 16b) were compared, differences were found on loading response (13% to 38% of the support phase) and terminal stance to pre swing phases (79% to 100% of the support phase). Differences between AS and NAS (Figure 16c) were found in the mid stance phase (45% to 60% of the support phase).

The shear forces are higher near the initial contact, loading response and terminal stance-to-pre swing phases in the CG COF curve; this pattern is not the same for the stroke group. The main differences between the stroke patients and the control group is that both AS and LAS performed lower shear forces during the loading response and terminal-to-pre swing phases. During these phases, the lower the friction was the higher was the risk of falling. Moreover, the AS group performed higher COF values in the mid stance than the LAS group and CG. In this case, the higher the friction, the higher was the risk of tripping.

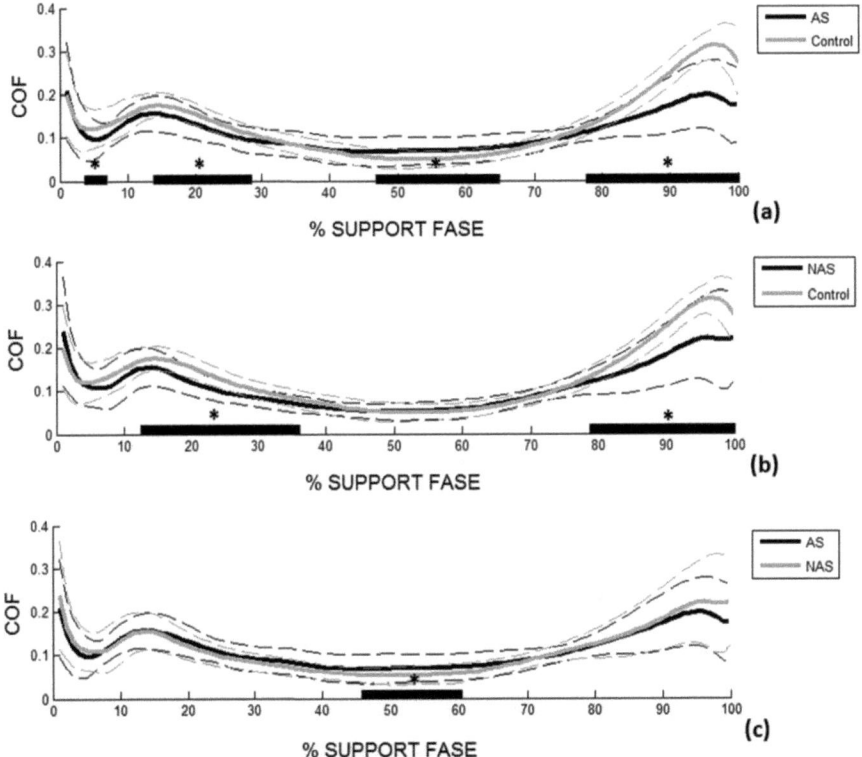

Figure 16. COF curve's mean and standard deviation in the comparisons between: (a) Stroke affected side (black solid line – mean, and black dashed line - standard deviation) and Control Group (grey line – mean, and grey dashed line - standard deviation); (b) Stroke non-affected side (black solid line – mean, and black dashed line - standard deviation) and Control Group (grey line – mean, and grey dashed line - standard deviation); and, (c) Stroke affected side (grey solid line – mean, and grey dashed line - standard deviation) and Stroke non-affected side (black solid line – mean, and black dashed line - standard deviation). The bars and asterisks on the x-axes indicate the moments of the support phase that presented significant differences (P ≤ 0.05) between the groups. Legend: AS = Stroke Group Affected Side; LAS = Stroke Group Less Affected Side; Control = Control Group; %SUPPORT PHASE = normalized by the percentage of the support phase.

5.4. Discussion

This study compared the gait of stroke patients and healthy age matched peers in an effort to quantify differences that may be predisposing the stroke population to falls.

When analyzing the instantaneous COF curves, it was noted that in normal gait patients the COF were higher than the stroke group near to the loading response and terminal stance phases. During these phases, the COF was actually higher when compared to the other stance phases, to firstly permit the deceleration phase for the loading acceptance and secondly the acceleration phase for guaranteeing the gait progression. It permits the right grip and consequently the transmission of the developed forces to the kinematic chain, reducing the slipping and the risk of falls. The loading response and the terminal stance are the critical phases in which slips often occur: the lower the friction is in these phases, the higher is the slipping risk (Chang et al., 2012; Redfern et al., 2001).

The analysis of the COF curves of the pathological group – for both AS and LAS sides – have evidenced lower values of COF on the same phases, pointing out a diminished grip on deceleration and acceleration phases. It seems that the stroke group reduced the gait velocity and, consequently, reduced the necessary (required) COF to perform the gait safely. In normal gait, once the deceleration phase starts, the COF decreases and the inertia forces sustain the gait progression: in that phase, the mid-stance, the contribution of the shear forces decreases in order to invert the decelerated movement and prepare the following acceleration phase. Considering the COF curve of AS of stroke participants, the COF showed higher values on this phase, pointing out a greater grip and a constraint in the motion inversion: this behavior breaks the contralateral side swing (LAS) decreasing the smoothness and increasing the level of balance uncertainty. The comparison between AS and LAS evidenced a statistical difference on the COF values in the mid-stance: on this phase the calf muscle is at its maximum stretching (the ankle reaches the maximum dorsiflexion and the knee the maximum extension – Bensoussan et al., 2006) and spasticity (Olney et al., 1991; Winter, 1983a) probably playing an important role in the progression constraint in AS.

Moreover, when compared to the control group, the stroke group AS and LAS presented higher V_1nor and P_2nor. Once these variables were normalized by the walking velocity, the results of this study show that in patients with stroke for the AS and LAS the mid stance and the terminal stance seems to be critical phases for slips incidence. This behavior can be explained by the stroke patients dropped foot. It is commonly described by kinematic deviations at the ankle – foot including forefoot or flat foot initial contact leading to reduced stability during stance. Stroke related to ankle impairments causes inadequate dorsiflexion control during gait, including weakness of dorsiflexors, spasticity of plantar flexors, passive stiffness of the plantar flexors, and abnormal muscle coactivation (Lamontagne et al., 2002). Moreover, limited ankle dorsiflexion and knee flexion during swing on AS often result in the use of compensatory strategies (i.e. pelvic hiking and circunduction) to achieve foot clearance (Chen et al., 2005; Kerrigan et al., 2001; Lindquist et al., 2007).

5.5. Conclusion

The stroke group have reduced the COF to perform the gait safely, what is probably related to compensatory strategies due to the altered AS motion during swing. The COF normalized by the walking velocity can be useful in predicting the real fall propensity of a stroke patient and to develop more effective therapy for the gait improvement. Moreover, the normalized COF shows that the mid stance and the terminal stance are phases of critical importance in determining if the frictional capabilities of the foot/floor interface to prevent slips in Stroke patients.

Chapter 6. The coefficient of friction during gait correlates with functional scales of Parkinson's Disease.

The Chapter 5 presented that persons with stroke present a characteristic COF curve pattern when compared with the aged matched control group. Does the COF curve also have a characteristic pattern in persons with Parkinson's Disease (PD)? The Chapter 6 were designed to characterize the COF curves of individuals with PD in barefoot gait and to analyze the possible correlations of this variable with the most used functional scales for the clinical evaluation of this disease, i.e., 6 Minutes Walk Test (6MW); the Timed Up & Go Test (TUG); the Unified Parkinson's Disease Rating Scale (UPDRS); and the Hoehn and Yahr scale (HY).

6.1. Introduction

Parkinsonian gait is marked by postural instability, small shuffling steps characterized by free ambulation with reduced stride length and walking speed, increases in double support duration and cadence (Morris et al., 2005; Morris et al., 2001; Morris et al., 1996; Morris et al, 1998; Morris et al, 1994); and difficulty freezing during goal-oriented gait tasks (Pieruccini-Faria et al., 2014). Furthermore, while walking, PD patients exhibit flat foot strikes in which the entire foot is placed on the ground at the same time, and they exhibit reduced foot lifting during the swing phase of gait, which produces reduced toe clearance. Although the literature contains many studies that have characterized Parkinson gait, particularly in terms of spatio-temporal and kinematic gait patterns, ground reaction forces and specifically the required coefficient of friction (RCOF) have not been sufficiently analyzed.

Thus, the characterization of the COF curves of PD patients and the correlations between specific COF areas and the most common used functional scales can provide some information about the influence of COF and the incidence of falls in this population. The most commonly used functional scales in PD are the following: the Six-Minute Walk Test (6MW), which is used to measure the maximum distance that a person can walk in 6 minutes (Steffen et al., 2002); the Timed Up & Go Test (TUG), which is a clinical measure of the balance of elderly people and is scored on an ordinal scale from 1 to 5 based on an observer's perception of the performer's risk of falling during the test (Rockwood et al., 2000; Steffen et al., 2002); the Unified Parkinson's Disease Rating Scale (UPDRS), which is a scale that is used to monitor PD-related disability and impairment (Song et al., 2009); and the Hoehn and Yahr scale (HY), which is a commonly used system for describing how the symptoms of Parkinson's disease progress (Hoehn and Yahr, 1967).

Our aims were to characterize the COF curves of patients with PD during barefoot gait and to analyse the possible correlations of this variable with the outcomes of the most commonly used functional scales for the evaluation of PD; i.e., the HY, UPDRS, TUG and 6MW.

6.2. Methods

6.2.1. Participants

The Parkinson group (PD) consisted of 22 patients affected by Parkinson's disease (9 females and 13 males). The average characteristics of the PD group were the following: age = 67.22±6.70 years; body mass = 76.5±18.83 kg; height = 161.59±11.01 m; UPDRS = 45.92±28.68; and H&Y = 2.76±0,788. PD was diagnosed based on clinical criteria (Gelb et al., 1999; Nutt and Wooten, 2005), dopamine transporter (DaT) scans and/or magnetic resonance imaging. The patients were similar in terms of disease duration and were also free of peripheral sensory neuropathy and other disorders based on their reported histories, symptoms, physical examinations and routine tests. Patients with liver, kidney, lung, or heart disease, diabetes or other causes of autonomic dysfunction were not included in the study.

The control group (CG) consisted of 22 healthy adults (9 females and 13 males) with the following average characteristics: age = 66.27±6 years; body mass = 73.22±11.45 kg; and height = 164.81± 10.10 m.

6.2.2. Data Collection

The data collection of this study was held at the Gait Analysis Lab, ICRSS San Raffaele Pisana, Rome, Italy. All tests of the PD patients was performed during the ON phase during their best motor conditions approximately 90 minutes after the first dose of levodopa in the morning.

6.2.3. Clinical assessments

Trained professionals performed all of the instrumental and clinical assessments. The clinical and instrumental outcomes were assessed using valid and reliable tools for PD that included the following: the Hoehn and Yahr scale (HY), the Unified Parkinson's Disease Rating Scale (UPDRS), the Timed Up & Go Test (TUG), and the Six-Minute Walk Test (6MW).

6.2.4. Experimental Procedures for motion analysis

The participant was directed to walk barefoot at a self-selected speed along a pathway covered by an experimental flooring that went over two force platforms (Kistler 9286BA) that were embedded in the floor of the data collection room. These platforms collected data at a frequency of 500 Hz. The participants were aware of the positions of the force plates. A single trial was performed.

Data acquisition was performed using a Smartanalyser (BTS, Italy). The raw kinetic data were filtered using a 2nd-order low-pass digital Butterworth filter with a cut-off frequency of 10 Hz. An algorithm developed in Matlab was used to filter the raw data and to calculate the dependent variables.

The ground reaction force data from the force plates were normalized by the subjects' body weights and are expressed as percentages of the support phase (%SP). The COF curve was calculated as described in Equation 1 (see Chapter 1).

Comparisons of the COF curves of the PD group with those of the control group revealed differences during the loading response, midstance and terminal stance phases. As shown in Figure 1, the COF patterns of the PD patients were characterized by diminished values during the loading response and terminal stance phases and increased values during the midstance phase. To quantify these behaviours, the areas of the curves of each patient with PD curve and the average curves of the CG were calculated as illustrated in Figure 17 and described in Equation 5.

$$Area = \int_b^a [f(x) - g(x)]\, dx \tag{5}$$

where $f(x)$ is the average COF curve of the CG, and $g(x)$ indicates the COF curve of each patient with PD.

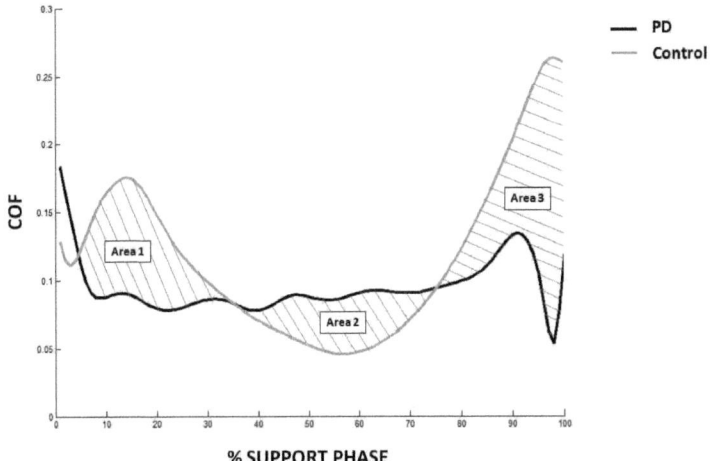

Figure 17.Illustrations of an example of one PD COF curve (black line) and the average curve for all CG (grey line) and the 3 phases were the area between the curves were calculated.

6.2.5. Statistical Analysis

For the statistical analyses, the data were first tested for normality with the Kolmoronov-Smirnov test. Because all of the behavioural data exhibited normal distributions, parametric statistics were applied. First, one-way ANOVAs ($\alpha \leq 0.05$) were applied to compare the anthropometric data (i.e., age, body mass and height) between the PD group and the CG. Furthermore, this test was applied to compare the differences between the right and left lower limbs of the PD group and the CG. Because no significant differences were found between the right and left limbs, the left limb was selected to represent the CG and PD bodies for all curve comparisons.

Comparisons between the mean COF curves of the PD patients and the CG were performed with two-sample T-tests ($\alpha \leq 0.05$) that were applied to every 1% of the gait cycle. Next, Pearson's correlations ($\alpha \leq 0.05$) were used to assess the associations between the COF curve areas and the outcomes of the following functional scales: the Hoehn and Yahr Scale (HY), the Unified Parkinson's Disease Rating Scale (UPDRS), the Timed Up & Go Test (TUG), and the Six-Minute Walk Test (6MW). According to Taylor (1999), the correlations were interpreted as follows: 0.9 to 1 indicated a very high correlation; 0.7 to 0.9 indicated a high correlation; 0.5 to 0.7 indicated a moderate correlation; 0.3 to 0.5 indicated a low correlation; and 0 to 0.3 indicated little to no correlation. All tests were two-tailed. SPSS (version 19) was used to perform all statistical analyses.

6.3. Results

A one-way ANOVA revealed no significant differences between the subjects with Parkinson's and the control group in terms of age ($F_{1,41}=0.272$; $p=0.605$), body mass ($F_{1,41}=0.485$; $p=0.490$) or height ($F_{1,19}=1.026$; $p=0.371$).

The COF curve analyses highlighted the following three phases during the support phase in which the Parkinson's patients exhibited alterations compared to the control group: during the loading response phase (10% to 31% of the support phase); during the midstance phase (45% to 71% of the

56

support phase), and during the terminal stance phase (82% to 95% of the support phase). Figure 18 illustrates these results.

The COFs were higher near the loading response and terminal stance phases in the CG, and this pattern was not observed in the PD group. The patients with PD exhibited lower COF values during the loading response and terminal stance phases compared to those exhibited by the CG.

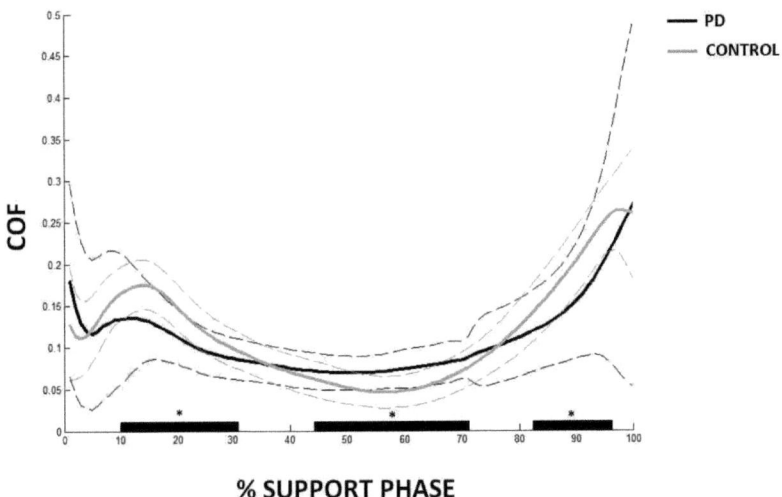

% SUPPORT PHASE

Figure 18. Mean and standard deviation of COF curve of the Parkinson Group (black solid line – mean, and black dashed line - standard deviation) and Control Group (grey line – mean, and grey dashed line - standard deviation. The bars and asterisks on the x-axes indicate the moments of the support phase that presented significant differences (P ≤ 0.05) between the PD and Control Group curves. Legend: PD = Parkinson Disease; Control = Control Group; %SUPPORT PHASE = normalized by the percentage of the support phase.

A significant and very high positive correlation was observed between Area 1 and the TUG outcomes ($\rho = 0.903$). Furthermore, a significant moderate positive correlation was found between Area 1 and the UPDRS1 ($\rho = 0.505$). Moreover, Area 1 and the 6MW (R = 0.672) exhibited a significant moderate negative correlation. Moderate positive significant correlations of Area 2 with the UPDRS$_2$ ($\rho = 0.515$) and UPDRS$_4$ ($\rho = 0.512$) were also observed. Table 6 illustrates all of these results.

Table 6. COF area and contact time in PD patients Correlation (Pearson Test – P $\leq$ 0.05) with the Functional Scales.

VARIABLES		Area$_1$	Area$_2$	Area$_3$
UPDRStotal	ρ	0.077	0.043	-0.065
	P	0.755	0.862	0.791
UPDRS$_1$ – Mentation, behavior and Mood	ρ	*0.505*	0.345	0.059
	P	*0.046*	0.191	0.827
UPDRS$_2$ – Activities and Daily Living	ρ	0.451	*0.515*	0.040
	P	0.080	*0.041*	0.882
UPDRS$_3$ – Motor Examination	ρ	0.488	0.105	-0.106
	P	0.055	0.699	0.696
UPDRS$_4$ – Complications of Therapy	ρ	-0.050	*0.512*	-0.179
	P	0.853	*0.043*	0.507
H&Y	ρ	0.249	0.461	0.115
	P	0.370	0.084	0.682
TUG	ρ	*0.903*	0.368	-0.035
	P	*0.0001*	0.161	0.896
6MW	ρ	*-0.672*	-0.095	-0.029
	P	*0.004*	0.726	0.914

6.4. Discussion

This study aimed to characterize the COF curves of patients with PD in the ON levodopa stage during gait and to evaluate the relationships between this index and functional scales.

When the COF curves of the PD groups were compared to those of the CG, the PD patients exhibited lower COFs during the loading response and terminal stance phases. This behaviour might be explained by the flat foot contact that has been observed during parkinsonian gait (Morris et al., 2005; Morris et al., 2001; Morris et al., 1996; Morris et al, 1998; Morris et al, 1994) and is likely related to the need to increase safety margins (Morris et al., 2005; Morris et al., 2001). Another possible explanation is related to the typical speed reductions of PD subjects that have previously been reported (Morris et al., 2005; Morris et al., 2001; Morris et al., 1996; Morris et al, 1998; Morris et al, 1994). Both of these effects, among others, might have contributed to the kinematical and dynamical alterations in the gait patterns of the PD patients that were revealed through examination of the COF curves. It would be interesting to determine the particular contribution of each effect on future studies.

A very high correlation was observed between Area 1 and the TUG in which higher Area 1 COFs were associated with increased times required to perform the TUG. Turning is an essential part of goal-directed locomotion that people engage in daily (Stack et al., 1994). However, turning difficulty is a common problem for people with PD (Stack et al., 1994). A previous study noted that more than 50% of patients with PD have difficulty turning that can lead to falls (Stack et al., 1994). Mak and Pang (2009) noted that the TUG test can be used to distinguish fallers from non-fallers; longer a TUG time (16 seconds) is independently associated with an increased risk of falls in patients with PD.

Besides, the Area 1 (the area that corresponds to the loading response period) is higher as the time to perform the Six Minutes Walking Test in PD patients is increased. It seems that the COF in loading response phase for PD patients is influenced by the gait velocity.

Moreover, the area during the loading response (Area 1) increased with the time required to perform the Six-Minute Walking Test in the patients with PD. It seems that the COF during the loading response phase was influenced by gait velocity in the PD patients. Moreover, in the loading response phase, the patients with PD exhibited increases in Area 1 that scaled with increases in cognitive decline (UPDRS$_1$). Cognitive decline is another independent risk factor for falls (Herman et al., 2010; Mirelman et al., 2012; Amboni et al., 2013). Gait disorders and falls are more prevalent among demented patients than nondemented subjects, and there is a direct relationship between the severity of cognitive impairment and increased gait abnormalities (Amboni et al., 2013; van Iersel et al., 2014). Gait is no longer merely considered to be automated motor activity but is rather an activity that requires executive function, attention, motivation and judgment of external and internal cues (Yogev-Seligmann et al., 2008). Given these associations and the effects of cognitive impairment and gait abnormalities on functional independence, these findings highlight the multiple links between gait, cognitive function, COF and falls.

During the midstance phase, the PD patients exhibited higher COFs than did the CG subjects. Considering that the coefficient of rolling resistance is generally much smaller than the coefficient of sliding friction, this result suggests that parkinsonian gait involves a less efficient rolling mechanism during the midstance phase. Furthermore, these mechanisms (Area 2) were correlated with the activities of the daily living (UPDRS$_2$) and the complications of therapy (UPDRS$_4$) of the PD patients. The proposed approach of observing the COF during gait revealed a compromise between decreased efficiency in favour of increased safety during parkinsonian gait.

Because the shear forces are highest near the loading response and terminal stance phases (Chang et al., 2012), these are the moments at which slips occur most often. The initial contact seems to be the critical phase in which slips can result in falls in patients with Parkinson's disease. The loading response causes forward slips on the leading foot, whereas the terminal stance causes backward slips on the forepart of the sole, which can more easily be counteracted by stepping forward with the leading foot (Redfern et al., 2001). Thus, the friction that occurs during the loading response is critically important for determining whether the frictional capabilities of the foot/floor interface will be sufficient to prevent slips in Parkinson's disease patients. The results of this study indicate that more severely affected PD patients exhibit greater her COF area values during the loading response phase.

Finally, to better characterize the COFs during parkinsonian gait, future studies should compare this variable between the levodopa ON and OFF stages. This comparison would provide a dissociation of the effects of levodopa from the basic motor disorder and an explanation of the physiological (or pathophysiological) meanings of the COFs of patients with PD.

6.5. Conclusion

In conclusion, in patients with PD, the COFs exhibited a specific pattern of differences from those of the CG; during the loading response phase, the difference was well correlated with the TUG scale data, which identifies the risk of falls among patients with PD. This analysis represents an initial first attempt to evaluate a gait analysis parameter in terms of its utility in the prediction of the real fall propensity of patients with PD. Furthermore, the analysis of COF can be simply applied because the patient is not required to change clothes for the positioning of markers and is only required to be barefoot. Therefore, the patient can be evaluated more easily during both the OFF and ON medication stages.

Final Considerations

The aim of this thesis is to analyze the RCOF in normal and pathological gait.

The first point to take into consideration about this study is that the friction in all the four studies presented was analyzed in barefoot gait. The studies usually investigate the RCOF in patients who perform tasks with shoes on. Therefore, this is a novelty, which pointed out that in barefoot gait, differences in RCOF are noticed considering the flooring conditions, the pathology type, and also the patients' age and gender.

Secondly, all the four surfaces presented in the Third and Fourth chapters, presented safe coefficient of friction (ranging from 0.44-0.55) and are widely used in residences and public facilities. We have chosen this type of dry flooring trying to simulate in laboratorial environment the same type of flooring that is found at the participants' homes. Once previous studies have already shown that a big number of falls happen when older adults walk barefoot inside their own houses/familiar environment (Menz et al, 2005), especially when moving from one room to another, or leaving the shower room or the swimming pool area. However, only few studies have reported the relation among the RCOF during elderly barefoot gait and different types of indoor flooring. So, we tried to fill this gap. Moreover, at the best of our knowledge, the thesis's Fourth chapter is the first study to report the relation between hemibodies in dynamic friction variables of gait in people after stroke during the walking on different flooring types.

This thesis also shows other novelties in its Fifth and Sixth chapters, in which analysis of the RCOF curve presented different pattern in the hemiparetic and PD gait. This study represents an initial attempt to evaluate a gait analysis parameter that might be used to predict the real fall propensity of patients with stroke and PD.

Future investigations need to be designed to evaluate the pattern of the RCOF curves in other types of pathologies, as well as to investigate the real potential of this variable to detect the risk of fall in elderly and pathological populations.

The main contribution of this thesis in the movement analysis field is the simplicity to apply the methodology to calculate the RCOF, and, also to evaluate this variant. The RCOF is a very simple and efficient tool developed to characterize the normal and pathological gait; it might be used in the prediction of the real fall propensity of the elderly and patients with pathologies such as PD and Stroke. Moreover, the RCOF is an easy variable to interpret and might help physicians and health professionals to easily identify some gait alterations. Furthermore, the analysis of RCOF can be simply applied, once the patient is not required to change clothes for the positioning of markers. He or she is only required to stay barefoot. That encourages a freer walking performance by the patients and makes it easier to evaluate his or her performance before and after any kind of intervention.

References

Amboni M, Barone P, Hausdorff JM. Cognitive Contributions to Gait and Falls: Evidence and Implication. *Mov Disord* 2013; 28(11): 1520-33.

Ashburn A, Stack E, Pickering RM, Ward CD. A community-dwelling sample of people with Parkinson's disease: characteristics of fallers and non-fallers. *Age Ageing* 2001;30:47–52.

Bhushan B. Introduction to Tribology. Wiley-Interscience: Toranto-Ontario, 2002.

Bhushan B. Principles and Applications of Tribology. Wiley-Interscience, 1999.

Barbic F, Galli M, Vecchia LD, Canesi M, et al. Effects of mechanical stimulation of the feet on gait and cardiovascular autonomic control in Parkinson's disease. *J Appl Physiol* 2014; 116: 495–503.

Berg, Katherine; Wood-Dauphinėe, Sharon; Williams, J.I.; Gayton, David. "Measuring balance in the elderly: preliminary development of an instrument". *Physiotherapy Canada* 1989; 41 (6): 304–311.

Bensoussan L, Mesure S, Viton JM, Delarque A. Kinematic and kinetic asymmetries in hemiplegic patients' gait initiation patterns. *J Rehabil Med* 2006; 38:287–94.

Bloem BR, Grimbergen YA, Cramer M, Willemsen M, Zwinderman AH. Prospective assessment of falls in Parkinson's disease. *J Neurol* 2001; 248:950– 8.

Bloem BR, Grimbergen YA, van Dijk JG, Munneke M. The "posture second" strategy: a review of wrong priorities in Parkinson's disease. *J Neurol Sci* 2006; 248(1-2): 196-204.

Blum, Lisa; Korner-Bitensky, Nicol. "Usefulness of the Berg Balance Scale in Stroke Rehabilitation: A Systematic Review". *Phys Ther* 2008; 88 (5): 559–566.

Bogle Thorbahn LD, Newton RA, Chandler J. Use of the Berg balance test to predict falls in elderly persons. *Phys Ther* 1996; 76: 576–586.

Bohannon RW, Andrews AW. Correlation of knee extensor muscle torque and spasticity with gait speed in patients with stroke. *Arch Phys Med Rehabil* 1990; 71:330-3.

Bönig S. Experimental investigation to determine the standardized limit of the coefficient of friction for slip resistance during walking. Tesis. Department of Safety Technology, University of Wuppertal, Germany, 1996.

Bowden FP, Tabor D. The friction and Lubrication of Solids. Clarendon Press Oxford, 1964, Vol. 2

Buczek FL, Cavanagh PR, Kulakowski BT, Pradhan P. Slip resistance needs of the mobility disabled during level grade walking. In Gray BE, editor. Slips, Stumbles and Falls: Pedestrian Footwear and Surfaces. Philadelphia, PA: ASTM; 1990, 39-54.

Burnfield, JM, Powers, CM. Influence of age and gender of utilized coefficient of friction during walking at different speeds. In: Marpet MI, Sapienza MA, editors. Metrology of pedestrian locomotion and slip resistance, ASTM STP 1424. West Conshohocken: ASTM International; 2003, 3–16.

Burnfield JM, Tsai YJ, Powers CM. Comparison of utilized coefficient of friction requirements in older persons with and without a disability to younger persons during different walking tasks. In Proceedings of the 8th Annual meeting of the Gait and Clinical Movement Analysis Society; 2003, 99-100.

Bunterngchit Y, Lockhart T, Woldstad J, Smith J. Age related effects of transitional floor surfaces and obstruction of view on gait characteristics related to slips and falls. *Int J Ind Ergonom* 2000; 25:223–232.

Carmo AA, Kleiner AFR, Lobo da Costa PH, Barros RML. Three-dimensional kinematic analysis of upper and lower limb motion during gait of post-stroke patients. *Braz J Med Biol Res* 2012; 45(6): 537-545.

Cham R, Redfern MS. Lower extremity corrective reactions to slip events. *J Biomech* 2001;34:1439–45.

Chang W. The effects of surface roughness on dynamic friction between neolite and quarry tile. *Saf Sci* 1998; 29 (2): 89-105.

Chang WR. The effects of surface roughness on the measurement of slip resistance. *Int J Ind Ergon* 1999; 24 (3), 299-313.

Chang WR. The effects of filtering process on surface parameters and their correlation with the measured friction, part II: porcelain tile. *Saf Sci* 2000; 36 (1), 35-47.

Chang WR, Matz S. The effect of filtering processes on surface roughness parameters and their correlation with the measured friction, part I: quarry tiles. *Saf Sci* 2000; 36 (1), 19-33.

Chang WR. The effects of surface roughness and contaminant on the dynamic friction of porcelain tile. *Appl Ergon* 2001; 32 (2), 173-184.

Chang WR. The effects of surface roughness and contaminants on the dynamic friction between porcelain tile and vulcanized rubber. *Saf Sci* 2002; 40 (7-8), 577-591.

Chang WR, Kim IJ, Manning DP, Bunterngchit Y. The role of surface roughness in the measurement of slipperiness. *Ergonomics* 2001; 44 (13), 1200-1216.

Chang WR, Groè Nqvist R, Leclercq S, Brungraber RJ, Mattke U, Strandberg L, Thorpe SC, Myung R, Makkonen L, Courtney TK. The role of friction in the measurement of slipperiness, Part 2: Survey of friction measurement devices, *Ergonomics* 2001; 44, 1233-1261.

Chang WR, Chang CC, Matz S. Comparison of different methods to extract the required coefficient of friction for level walking. *Ergonomics* 2012; 55(3):308-315.

Chao EY, Laughman RK, Schneider E, Stauffer R. Normative data of knee joint motion and ground reaction forces in adult level walking. *J Biomech* 1983; 16, 219-233.

Chen C, Patten C, Kothari DH. Gait differences between individuals with post-stroke hemiparesis and non-disabled controls at matched speeds. *Gait Posture* 2005; 22:51-6.

Damiano AM, Snyder C, Strausser B, Willian MK. A review of health-related quality-of-life concepts and measures for Parkinson's disease. *Qual Life Res* 1999; 8:235–43.

Dickinson JI, Shroyer JL, Elias JW, Hutton JT, Gentry GM. The Effect of Selected Residential Carpet and Pad on the Balance of Healthy Older Adults. *Env Behav March* 2001; 33, 279-295.

Dorsey ER, Constantinescu R, Thompson JP et al. Projected number of people with Parkinson disease in the most populous nations, 2005 through 2030. *Neurology* 2007; 68:384–6.

Durá JV, Alcántara E, Zamora T, Balaguer E, Rosa D. Identification of floor friction safety level for public buildings considering mobility disabled people needs. *Safety Sci* 2005; 43:407-423.

Ekkebus CF, Killey W. Measurement of safe walkway surfaces. Soaps/Cosmetics/Chemical Specialties 1973; February:40–45.

Ferber R, McClay DI, Williams DS. Gender differences in lower extremity mechanics during running. *Clin Biomech* 2003; 18, 350–7.

Flansbjer UB, Holmbäck AM, Downham D, Patten C, Lexell J: Reliability of gait performance tests in men and women with hemiparesis after stroke. *J Rehab Med* 2005; 37:75-82.

Folstein MF, Folstein SE, McHugh PR. Mini-mental state: a practical method for grading the cognitive state of patients for the clinician". *J Psych Research* 1975; 12 (3): 189–98.

Fuhrer H, Kupsch A, Hälbig TD, Kopp UA, Scherer P, Gruber D. Levodopa inhibits habit-learning in Parkinson's disease. *J Neural Transm* 2014; 121:147–151.

Evers SM, Struijs JN, Ament AJ, van Genugten ML, Jager JC, van den Bos GA: International comparison of stroke cost studies. *Stroke* 2004, 35:1209-1215.

Gelb DJ, Oliver E, Gilman S. Diagnostic criteria for Parkinson disease. *Arch Neurol* 1999; 56: 33–39.

Gladstone DJ, Danells CJ, Black SE. The fugl-meyer assessment of motor recovery after stroke: a critical review of its measurement properties. *Neurorehabil Neural Repair* 2002; 16(3):232-40.

Graafmans WC, Ooms ME, Hofstee HMA. Falls in the elderly: a prospective study of risk factors and risk profiles. *Am J Epidemiol*. 1996; 143:1129–1136.

Gray P, Hildebrand K. Fall risk factors in Parkinson's disease. *J Neurosci Nurs* 2000; 32:222–8.

Grönqvist R, Roine J, Järvinen E, Korhonen E. An apparatus and a method for determining the slip resistance of shoes and floors by simulation of human foot motions. *Ergonomics* 1999; 32(8): 10-15.

Guttman, M., Kish, S. J., & Furukawa, Y. Current concepts in the diagnosis and management of Parkinson's disease. *Cmaj* 2003; 168(3), 293-301.

Haas CT, Buhlmann A, Turbanski, S, Schmidtbleicher D. Proprioceptive and sensorimotor performance in Parkinson's disease. *Res Sports Med* 2006; 14(4), 273-287.

Hanson JP, Redfern MS, Mazumdar M. Predicting slips and falls considering required and available friction. *Ergonomics* 1999; 42(12):1619–33.

Harris JE, Eng JJ, Marigold DS, Tokuno CD, Louis CL. Relationship of Balance and Mobility to Fall Incidence in People With Chronic Stroke. *Phys Ther* 2005; 85:150-158.

Haynes CA, Lockhart TE. Evaluation of Gait and Slip Parameters for Adults with Intellectual Disability. *J Biomech* 2012; 45(14): 2337–2341.

Herman T, Mirelman A, Giladi N, Schweiger A, Hausdorff JM. Executive control deficits as a prodrome to falls in healthy older adults: a prospective study linking thinking, walking, and falling. *J Gerontol A Biol Sci Med Sci* 2010; 65:1086–1092.

Hoehn MM, Yahr MD. Parkinsonism: onset, progression, and mortality. Neurology 1967; 17:427–42.

Holder-Powell H, Rutherford O. Unilateral lower-limb musculoskeletal injury: Its long term effect on balance. *Arch Phys Med Rehabil* 2000; 81: 265–268.

Hyndman D, Ashburn A, Stack E. Fall events among people with stroke living in the community: circumstances of falls and characteristics of fallers. *Arch Phys Med Rehabil* 2002; 83:165–170.

Hyndman D, Ashburn A. People with stroke living in the community: attention deficits, balance, ADL ability, and falls. *Disabil Rehabil* 2003; 25:817– 822.

Jenkins ME, Almeida QJ, Spaulding J, van Oostveen RB, et al. Plantar cutaneous sensory stimulation improves single-limb support time, and EMG activation patterns among individuals with Parkinson's disease. *Parkinsonism Relat Disord* 2009; 15 697–702.

Israelachvili JN. Surface Forces and Microrheology of Molecularly Thin Liquid Films, in: Handbook of Micro/Nanotribology; B. Bushan, Ed., CRC Press, 1995, pp. 267-319.

Johnson, AA. The impact of exercise rehabilitation and physical activity on the management of Parkinson's disease. *Geriatr Aging* 2007; 10: 318-321.

Jorgensen L, Engstad T, Jacobsen BK. Higher incidence of falls in long-term stroke survivors than in population controls: depressive symptoms predict falls after stroke. *Stroke* 2002; 33:542–547.

Kavounoudias A, Roll R, Roll JP. The plantar sole is a dynamometric map for human balance control. *Neuroreport* 1998; 9:3247–52.

Kemmlert K, Lundholm L. Slips, trips and falls in different work groups—with reference to age and from a preventive perspective. *Appl Ergon* 2001; 32, 149–153.

Kerrigan DC, Karvosky ME, Riley PO: Spastic paretic stiff-legged gait: joint kinetics. *Am J Phys Med Rehabil* 2001; 80: 244–9.

Kim IJ, Smith R. Observation of the floor surface topography changes in pedestrian slip resistance measurements. *Int J Ind Ergon* 2000; 6 (6), 581-601.

Kim IJ, Smith R. A critical analysis of the relationship between shoeefloor wear and pedestrian/walkway slip resistance. In: Marpet, M., Sapienza, M. (Eds.), Metrology of Pedestrian Locomotion and Slip Resistance. ASTM International, 2003, 33-48.

Kim IJ, Smith R, Nagata H. Microscopic observations of the progressive wear on the shoe surfaces that affect the slip resistance characteristics. *Int J Ind Ergon* 2001; 28 (1), 17-29.

Kim IJ. Development of a new analyzing model for quantifying pedestrian slip resistance characteristics: Part I - Basic concepts and theories. *Int J Ind Ergon* 2004a; 33 (5), 395-401.

Kim IJ. Development of a new analyzing model for quantifying pedestrian slip resistance characteristics: Part II - Experiments and validations. *Int J Ind Ergon* 2004b; 33 (5), 403-414.

Kim IJ, Nagata H. Nature of the Shoe Wear: Its Uniqueness, Complexity and Effects on Slip Resistance Properties. *Contemporary Ergonomics* 2008. Taylor & Francis, 2008a; pp. 728-734.

Kim IJ, Nagata H. Research on slip resistance measurements e a new challenge. *Ind Health* 2008b, 46, 68-78.

Kim S, Lockhart T, Yoon Y. Relationship between age-related gait adaptations and required coefficient of friction. *Safety Sci* 2005; 43:425–436.

Kim S, Lockhart T. Gait asymmetry—Factors influencing slip severity and tendency among older adults. Paper presented at the HFES conference, San Francisco, CA, 2006.

Kim S, Nagata IH. Research on slip resistance measurement - A new challenge. *Ind Health* 2008; 46, 66–76

Kim I, Hsio H, Simeonov P. Functional levels of floor surface roughness for the prevention of slips and falls: clean-and-dry and soapsuds-covered wet surfaces. Applied *Ergonomics* 2013; 44: 58-64.

Klit H, Finnerup NB, Jensen TS. Central post-stroke pain: clinical characteristics, pathophysiology, and management. *Lancet* Neurol 8:857-868, 2009.

Koozekanani SH, Balmaseda Jr., Fatehi MT, Lowney ED. Ground reaction forces during ambulation in Parkinsonism: pilot study. *Arch Phys Med Rehabil* 1987; 68: 28-30.

Korpelainen JT, Sotaniemi KA, Myllyla VV. Autonomic nervous system disorders in stroke. *Clin Auton Res* 1999; 9:325-333.

Kwakkel G, Kollen BJ, Wagenaar RC. Therapy Impact on Functional Recovery in Stroke Rehabilitation: A critical review of the literature. *Physiotherapy* 1999; 85:377-391.

Labyt E, Devos D, Bourriez JL, Cassim F, Destee A, Guieu JD. Motor preparation is more impaired in Parkinson's disease when sensorimotor integration is involved. *Clin Neurophysiol* 2003; 114:2423–33.

Lach HW. Incidence and Risk Factors for Developing Fear of Falling in Older Adults. *Public Health Nurs* 2005; 22(1): 45—52.

Lamb SE, Ferrucci L, Volapto S. Risk factors for falling in home-dwelling older women with stroke: the women's health and aging study. *Stroke* 2003; 34:494 –501.

Layne LA, Pollack KM. Nonfatal occupational injuries from slips, trips, and falls among older workers treated in hospital emergency departments, United States 1998. *Am J Ind Med* 2004; 46 (1), 32–41.

Leamon TB, Murphy PL. Occupational slips and falls: more than a trivial problem. *Ergonomics* 1995; 38 (3), 487–498.

Lewis GN, Byblow WD. Altered sensorimotor integration in Parkinson's disease. *Brain* 2002; 125:2089–99.

Li Y, Wang W, Crompton RH, Gunther MM. Free vertical moments and transverse forces in human walking and their role in relation to arm-swing. *J Exp Biol* 2011; 204, 47–58.

Lindquist AR, Prado CL, Barros RM, Mattioli R, da Costa PH, Salvini TF: Gait training combining partial body-weight support, a treadmill, and functional electrical stimulation: effects on poststroke gait. *Phys Ther* 2007; 87:1144-1154.

Lockhart TE. The ability of elderly people to traverse slippery walking surfaces. Proceedings of the Human Factors and Ergonomics Society 41st Annual Meeting. (Santa Monica, CA: Human Factors and Ergonomics Societies) 1997; 1: 125 – 129.

Lockhart TE, Woldstad JC, Smith JL. Assessment of slip severity among different age groups. Paper presented at the meeting of the American Society for Testing and Materials; West Conshohocken, PA. 2002.

Lockhart TE, Woldstad JC, Smith JL. Effects of age-related gait changes on biomechanics of slips and falls. *Ergonomics* 2003; 46:1136–1160.

Lockhart T, Kim S, Kapur R, Jarrott S. Evaluation of Gait Characteristics and Ground Reaction Forces in Cognitively Declined Older Adults With an Emphasis on Slip-Induced Falls. *Assist Technol* 2009; 21(4): 188–195.

Mak MK, Pang MY. Balance confidence and functional mobility are independently associated with falls in people with Parkinson's disease. J Neurol 2009; 256: 742–749.

Mayer M: Clinical neurokinesiology of spastic gait. Bratislavské lekárske listy 2002, 103:3-11.

Mayo NE, Korner-Bitensky NA, Becker R. Recovery time of independent function post-stroke. *Am J Phys Med Rehabil* 1991; 70:5–12.

Mayo NE, Wood-Dauphinee S, Ahmed S, Gordon C, Higgins J, McEwen S, Salbach N, Disablement following stroke. *Disabil Rehabil* 1999; 21(5):258–268.

Menz BM, Morris ME, Lord SR. Footwear characteristics and risk of indoor and outdoor falls in older people. *Gerontology* 2006; 52:174–180.

Miller JM. "Slippery" work Surfaces: Towards a Performance Definition and Quantitative Coefficient of Friction Criteria. *J Safety Res* 1983; 14(4), 145-158.

Mirelman A, Herman T, Brozgol M. Executive function and falls in older adults: new findings from a five-year prospective study link fall risk to cognition. *PLoS One* 2012; 7:402-407.

Mizrahi J, Susak Z, Heller L, Najenson T. Variation of time-distance parameters of the stride as related to clinical gait improvement in hemiplegics. *Scand J Rehabil Med* 1982; 14:133-40.

Mizuno Y, Kumagai M, Mattessich SM, Elias JJ, Ramrattan N, Cosgarea AJ, Chao EJ. Q-angle influences tibiofemoral and patellofemoral kinematics. *J Orthop Res* 2001; 19, 834–840.

Morita S, Yamamoto H, Furuya K. Gait analysis of hemiplegic patients by measurement of ground reaction force. *Scand J Rehabil Med* 1995; 27:37-42.

Morris ME, Iansek R, McGinley J, Matyas T, Huxham F. Three-Dimensional Gait Biomechanics in Parkinson's Disease: Evidence for a Centrally Mediated Amplitude Regulation Disorder. *Mov Disord* 2005; 20(1): 40–50.

Morris ME, Huxham F, McGinley J, Dodd K, Iansek R. The biomechanics and motor control of gait in Parkinson's disease. *Clin Biomech* 2001; 16: 459–470.

Morris M, Iansek R, Matyas T, Summers J. Abnormalities in the stride length-cadence relation in parkinsonian gait. *Mov Disord* 1998;13:61– 69.

Morris ME, Iansek R, Matyas TA, Summers JJ. Stride length regulation in Parkinson's disease. Normalization strategies and underlying mechanisms. *Brain* 1996; 119(2):551–568.

Morris ME, Iansek R, Matyas TA, Summers JJ. The pathogenesis of gait hypokinesia in Parkinson's disease. *Brain* 1994; 117(5):1169 –1181.

Nadeau S, Arsenault AB, Gravel D, Bourbonnais D. Analysis of the clinical factors determining natural and maximal gait speeds in adults with a stroke. *Am J Phys Med Rehabil* 1999; 78:123-30.

Nutt JG, Wooten GF. Clinical practice. Diagnosis and initial management of Parkinson's disease. *N Engl J Med* 353: 1021–1027, 2005.

Okazaki VHA, Teixeira LA, Rodacki ALF. Eficácia da Análise Residual Para Determinar a Intensidade do Filtro na Cinemática. In: XII Congresso Brasileiro de Biomecânica, 2007, São Pedro-SP, Brasil. XII Congresso Brasileiro de Biomecânica, 2007. v. XII. p. 1-5.

Olney SJ, Griffin MP, Monga TN, McBride ID. Work and power in gait of stroke patients. *Arch Phys Med Rehabil* 1991; 72:309–14.

O'Loughlin JL, Boivin JF, Robitaille Y. Falls among the elderly: distinguishing indoor and outdoor risk factors in Canada. *BMC Health Services Ressearch* 1994; 48:488–489.

Persson BNJ. Sliding Friction - Physical Principles and Applications, 2 ed.; Springer Heidelberg, 2000, Vol. 1.

Perry J. Gait analysis: normal and pathological function. NJ: SLACK Inc.; 1992. J. Perry, M. Garrett, J. K. Gronley, S. J. Mulroy, Classification of walking handicap in the stroke population. *Stroke* 1995; 26:982–989.

Perry SD. Evaluation of age-related plantar-surface insensitivity and onset age of advanced insensitivity in older adults using vibratory and touch sensation tests. *Neurosci Lett* 2006; 392:62–7.

Pieruccini-Faria F, Jones JA, Almeida QJ. Motor planning in Parkinson's disease patients experiencing freezing of gait: The influence of cognitive load when approaching obstacles. *Brain Cognition* 2014; 87:76–85.

Pratorius B, Kimmeskamp S, Milani TL. The sensitivity of the sole of the foot in patients with Morbus Parkinson. *Neurosci Lett* 2003;346:173–6.

Redfern MS, Dipasquale JD. Biomechanics of descending ramps. *Gait Posture* 19978; 6: 119- 125.

Redfern MS, Cham R, Gielo-Perczak K, Grönqvist R, Hirvonen M, Lanshammar H, Marpet. Biomechanics of Slips. *Ergonomics* 2001; 44(13):1138-1166.

Richardson JTE. Eta squared and partial eta squared as measures of effect size in educational research. *Rev Educ Res* 2011:6(2), 135-147.

Rockwood K, Awalt E, Carver D, MacKnight C. Feasibility and measurement properties of the functional reach and the timed up and go tests in the Canadian Study of Health and Aging. *J Gerontol A Biol Sci Med Sci* 2000; 55:M70 –M73.

Rossignol S, Dubuc R, Gossard JP: Dynamic sensorimotor interactions in locomotion. *Physiol Rev* 2006; 86:89.

Sadeghi H, Allard P, Prince F, Labelle H. Symmetry and limb dominance in able-bodies gait: a review. *Gait Posture* 2000; 12:34–45.

Salzma MD. Gait and balance disorders in older adults. *Am Fam Physician* 2010; 82(1):61-68.

Schaafsmaa JD, Giladia N, Balasha Y, Bartelsa AL, Gurevicha T, Hausdorff JM. Gait dynamics in Parkinson's disease: relationship to Parkinsonian features, falls and response to levodopa. *J Neurol Sci* 2003; 202:47– 53.

Schaechter JD. Motor rehabilitation and brain plasticity after hemiparetic stroke. *Prog Neurobiol* 2004, 73:61-72.

Schmidt H, Werner C, Bernhardt R, Hesse S, Krüger J. Gait rehabilitation machines based on programmable footplates. *J Neuroeng Rehabil* 2007; 4.

Seo J, Kim S. Asymmetrical slip propensity: required coefficient of friction. *J Neuroeng Rehabil* 2013a; 10:1-4.

Seo J, Kim S. Prevention of Potential Falls of Elderly Healthy Women: Gait Asymmetry. *Educ Gerontol* 2013b; 0: 1–15.

Silva-Smith AL, Kluge MA, LeCompte M, Snook A. Improving staff reports of falls in assisted living. *Clin Nurs Res* 2013; 22(4):448 –460.

Skelton D, Kennedy J, Rutherford O. Explosive power and asymmetry in leg muscle function in frequent fallers and non-fallers aged over 65. *Age Ageing* 2002; 31, 119–125.

Stack EL, Asburn AM, Jupp KE. Strategies used by people with Parkinson's disease who report difficulty turning. *Parkinsonism Relat Disord* 1994; 12: 87–92.

Steffen T, Hacker T, Mollinger L. Age-and gender-related test performance in community-dwelling elderly people: Six-Minute Walk Test, Berg Balance Scale, Timed Up & Go Test, and gait speeds. *Phys Ther* 2002;82:128 –137.

Stephens JM, Goldie PA. Walking speed on parquetry and carpet after stroke: effect of surface and retest reliability. *Clin Rehabil* 1999; 13:171–181.

Seo J, Kim S. Asymmetrical slip propensity: required coefficient of friction. *J Neuroeng Rehabil* 2013;10:1-4.

Shumway-Cook A, Woollacott M. Motor Control: theory and pratical applications. Baltimore: Willians & Wilkins; 1995.

Song J, Fisher BE, Petzinger G, Wu A, Gordon J, Salem GJ: The relationships between the UPDRS and lower extremity functional performance in persons with early parkinson's disease. *Neurorehabil Neural Repair* 2009, 23:657–661.

Steffen T, Hacker T, Mollinger L. Age-and gender-related test performance in community-dwelling elderly people: Six-Minute Walk Test, Berg Balance Scale, Timed Up & Go Test, and gait speeds. *Phys Ther* 2002; 82:128–137.

Taylor R. Interpretation of the Correlation Coefficient: A Basic Review. *JDMS* 1999; 1:35-39.

Teasall R, McRae M, Foley N, Bhardwaj A. The incidence and consequences of falls in stroke patients during inpatient rehabilitation: factors associated with high risk. *Arch Phys Med Rehabil* 2002;83: 329–333.

Templer, J. The Staircase: Studies of Hazards, Falls, and Safer Design. The MIT Press, Cambridge, Mass, 1992.

Titianova EB, Tarkka IM. Asymmetry in walking performance and postural sway in patients with chronic unilateral cerebral infarction. *J Rehabil Res Dev* 1995; 32:236-44.

Tsai, YJ, Powers, CM. The influence of footwear sole hardness on utilized coefficient of friction during walking. *Gait Posture 2009;* 30, 303–306.

Tsukruk VV, Bliznyuk VN, Hazel J, Visser D. Organic Molecular Films under Shear Forces: Fluid and Solid Langmuir Monolayers, Langmuir, 12, 1996, 4840-4849.

Twelves D, Perkins KS, Counsell C. Systematic review of incidence studies of Parkinson's disease. *Mov Disord* 2003; 18:19–31.

Ueno E, Yanagisawa N, Takami M. Gait disorders in Parkinsonism a study with floor reaction forces and EMG. *Adv Neurol* 1993; 60:414–418.

van Iersel MB, Hoefsloot W, Munneke M, Bloem BR, Olde Rikkert MG. Systematic review of quantitative clinical gait analysis in patients with dementia. *Z Gerontol Geriatr 2004*; 37:27–32.

Verma R, Arya KN, Sharma P, Garg RK. Understanding gait control in poststroke: Implications for management. *J Bodyw Mov Ther* 2010, 1-8.

Voncampenhausen S, Bornschein B, Wick R. Prevalence and incidence of Parkinson's disease in Europe. *Eur Neuropsychopharmacol* 2005; 15:473–90.

Wang TY, Lin SI. Sensitivity of plantar cutaneous sensation and postural stability. *Clin Biomech* 2008; 23:493–9.

Willmott M. The effect of vinyl floor surface and a carpet floor surface upon walking in elderly hospital patients. *Age Aging* 1986; 15, 199-120.

Winter DA. Biomechanical motor patterns in normal walking. *J Mot Behav* 1983a; 15:302–30.

Winter DA. Energy generation and absorption at the ankle and knee during fast, natural, and slow cadences. Clin Orthop Relat Res 1983b; 147–54.

Winter DA. Biomechanics and motor control of human movement. Wiley-Interscience: Toranto-Ontario, 1990.

Wirdefeldt K, Adami H, Cole, P, Trichopoulos D, Mandel J. Epidemiology and etiology of Parkinson's disease: a review of the evidence. *Eur J Epidemiol* 2011; 26:S1–S58.

World Health Organization. The World Health Report 2003: Shaping the future. Geneva: World Health Organization 2003.

Wood BH, Bilclough JA, Bowron A, Walker RW. Incidence and prediction of falls in Parkinson's disease: a prospective multidisciplinary study. *J Neurol Neurosurg Psychiatry* 2002;72:721–5.

Wyller TB, Kirkevold M. How does a cerebral stroke affect quality of life? Towards anadequate theoretical account. *Disabil Rehabil* 1999; 21:152–161.

Yogev-Seligmann G, Hausdorff JM, Giladi N. The role of executive function and attention in gait. *Mov Disord* 2008;23:329–342.

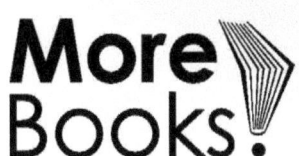
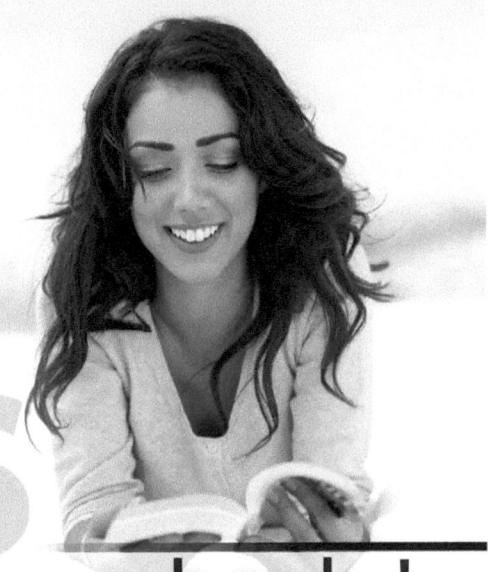 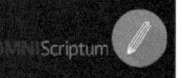

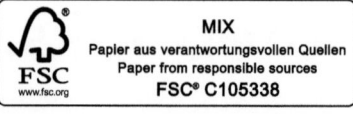